FLOURISH 2021 WRITERS, ET AL.

The Flourish Experience

THE POWER OF ADOPTEE HEALING IN COMMUNITY

Edited by: **DIANE SHIFFLETT**

ISBN: 979-8-9861628-0-5 (Paperback)

ISBN: 979-8-9861628-1-2 (Hardback)

ISBN: 979-8-9861628-3-6 (EBook)

Printed by Ingram Spark, in the United States of America.

First printing edition 2022

Publisher: The Flourish Experience

THE FLOURISH EXPERIENCE:
THE POWER OF ADOPTEE HEALING IN COMMUNITY

Dedication

WE DEDICATE THIS ANTHOLOGY to those who have felt silenced, ignored, or voiceless as adoptees. We write in memory of adoptees whose trauma led to death from suicide, addiction, loneliness or despair. We encourage fellow adoptees to find and create community to hold, validate and support them. May the experiences and art herein act as a beacon, guiding to a more compassionate future in which we are seen, heard, and valued as we are. A future in which all may thrive and flourish.

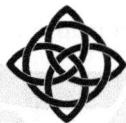

Foreword

PAM AND I WERE SITTING on her couch with paper and pens, looking to name a feeling. Since we couldn't do adoptee retreats in person because of Covid-19, we'd settled on the wild idea of having Zoom meetings once a week for an entire year, and now we had to think of what to call it.

The goal was to create a group with the intention of getting together in order to flower, bloom, expand, and break free of limiting beliefs. I drew flowers on the paper. We talked and I drew the sun, Earth, birds in flight. We wanted to create an environment where people could feel expansive, valuable, loved.

Pam said it first: Flourish.

We sat on the couch and repeated the word. The more we said it, the more we both liked how it sounded, the slide of the f and l; we liked that it was a verb, something you could do, and that it was also a noun, something you could be. The definitions were:

1. verb: (of a person, animal, or other living organism) grow or develop in a healthy or vigorous way, especially as the result of a particularly favorable environment.

2. noun: a bold or extravagant gesture or action, made especially to attract the attention of others.

3. noun: an instance of suddenly performing or developing in an impressively successful way.

We loved the words grow, develop, healthy, vigorous, favorable environment, bold, extravagant, attract, suddenly. How could you argue with impressively successful?

Flourish.

More than a year later, at the conclusion of the meetings, the groups were more than we'd imagined.

They were more magical, more dedicated, more complex, more confrontational, more extravagant. We saw demonstrations of despair, fury, love, connection, alienation, growth, hope, and friendship among so many other emotions and occurrences.

Flourish had become its own thing, a kind of strange family: people who had come to depend on each other being there every Wednesday night or Sunday morning. Adopted people sometimes find that depending on another can be very complicated, especially when there is a time the group will no longer meet after weeks and weeks of getting attached.

I thought a year would be enough for a group of adopted people to flourish, and while the growth and changes were remarkable, it also feels like in many ways the year was just a beginning, and so it is no surprise to see that many members of each group continue to meet weekly. I saw over the year, again and again, how much we need each other; I saw just how much community means to those who know what it is to feel alone.

We are courageous people, we adoptees. We want to flourish. We play hard. We cry hard. We laugh hard. We try.

Anne Heffron and Pam Cordano

Co-creators of Flourish (2020-2021)

January 31, 2022

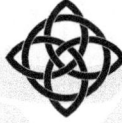

Introduction

ARE YOU AN ADOPTED PERSON? Have you spent much time with adopted people? Is someone you love an adopted person? Have you ever wondered what living life as an adopted person is like?

This book contains a collection of writings and artwork by a community of adopted people who participated in a class called Flourish. In 2021, more than thirty of us met for two hours once a week, every week, in two different classes, for the whole year, to explore healing through community and the joy and hard work of writing ourselves into the world. These pages are a window into our lives and experiences of adoption.

All of the people in class, including those who contributed to this book, are adopted persons. We live in different countries, hemispheres, seasons, and states of mind. Our home lives, childhoods, professions, and the circumstances of our adoption are different. We differ in age, gender, ancestry, religion, sexual preference. Some of us were published writers before joining the class, others had never written anything to be shared with another person, ever.

Through exploring our lived, adopted experiences within this diverse group of people, we found commonality and community. Each week we shared what we had lived through. We found that, although we felt alone in our pain, these life experiences are common for adopted people. We believe these experiences and the feelings of isolation can and should be improved. Adoption was not a single event and the effects of adoption on our lives cannot be overstated. This class helped us to put words to our feelings and experiences and see how to move forward.

We would not have been able to make those moves or write our truths without Pam Cordano and Anne Heffron. Pam gave freely of her wild spirit, her professional experience as a psychotherapist, and her uncanny ability to draw out vital sparks of meaning and growth even in what seemed to be the barest of gardens. The consummate writing teacher, Anne challenged us to find a way past our roadblocks and creatively reframe our lives through writing. Always asking us could we say more, be bigger, be louder, own our truth. We will always be thankful for their leadership, their truth, and their whole-hearted commitment to us and our class.

As you read the book you may notice there is no standard language of adoption. Birth mother, first mother, B-mother, adoptive mother, adopted mother, A-mother, mother can all be used in the same story. Every adopted person has their own way of expressing relationship. You may need to read for context to understand these relationships. Doing this may give you insight into the complexities, large and small, that many adopted persons live with.

Reunion in the context of adoption refers to finding and meeting one or more biological relatives, especially a birth parent. Reunion can be a roller coaster of emotions including joy, anger, dismay, disappointment, resentment, love and regret. When a biological family member chooses to end or may not be willing to start a relationship with the adopted person this is called secondary rejection and can be devastating. Not every adopted person is able to learn who their biological family of origin is. They may never meet their birth parents, know if they have siblings, or know anything at all about their medical history or heritage. They live with the pain of longing to meet someone who is biologically related, who shares inherited characteristics, or mirrors their expressions, feelings, or interests and knowing this is unlikely to happen.

Coming out of the fog is a phrase that has a particular meaning in the adoption community. It refers to recognizing and experiencing the grief and loss of relinquishment and abandonment and learning to live in the truth of what it means to be an adopted person. The pain, trauma, and intensely personal experience of coming out of the fog is difficult, if not impossible, to explain to someone who has no personal experience of being an adopted person. Finding supportive people and fellow adopted persons who do understand can make a world of difference.

We know that the people who best understand the experience of being adopted are the people who have lived it. And we believe that the best resource on the experience of being adopted are adopted people. If you are an adopted person feeling alone, we understand, each in our own ways. One of the ways we want to create space for you in our community is through this book. As such, the statements in this book are not meant to represent the lives, feelings, thoughts, or experiences of all adopted persons. For more information on the experience of being adopted, please see the resource list at the back of the book.

The authors' names in this volume offer another opportunity to consider the complexities of being part of and not part of different families, as well as owning or not owning, knowing or not knowing your personal story. The name each author has chosen reflects their personal choice. Some have chosen to use the name given by their adoptive family, others elected to use their birth name, and some have claimed a different name for themselves. Each chapter also includes a short biography of the author. The chapters are titled by author and their work following. A list of the monthly class topics and the writing prompts can be found at the end of the book.

The driving force behind this book was to both create a record of our time together and to say to other adopted people "You are not alone. We see you." After a year of hearing the commonalities at the root of our experiences as adopted persons, feeling the power of writing and sharing our truths, we recognize the potency and capacity for growth, healing and a greater sense of agency generated in community. Just as we shared them over a year together in Flourish, here we offer you our stories, thoughts, feelings and experiences to educate, inspire, spark discussion, and offer connection.

Here are some of the truths we hope to share with you:

- The voices of adopted people matter, including yours
- The feelings and experiences of adopted people are real and relevant, including yours
- We find belonging in this community of shared experiences, as could you
- Adoptees in community create powerful healing potential
- All adopted persons and their allies are welcome members of our shared community

What is a community of adopted persons committed to supporting each other and lifting our true voices? An ideal environment for healing and growth, a force elevating the visibility of the experiences of adopted persons, a place in which we can truly FLOURISH!

Join us! You can flourish, too! Just turn the page.

This book is a result of an adoptee community coming together to heal and grow. This book and the friendships formed through this experience could not have been possible without the connections made through Haley Radke and the *Adoptees On* podcast. All proceeds from this book will go to support *Adoptees*

On so that more adoptees can find their own Flourish family, a community of adoptees who "get it." *Adoptees On* is where incredible adopted people are willing to share their intimately personal stories about the impact adoption has had on their lives. People who were adopted can listen in and discover they are not alone on this journey.

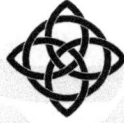

About the Artwork

THE BEAUTIFUL ARTWORK found in this book and on its cover was created by Flourish members Michelle Madsen Hinton, Francine J Bauer and Susie Stricker. The artwork was created in collaboration for the book to reflect our experience together. The original work and a limited release of prints were sold and auctioned in support of Saving Our Sisters (SOS), an advocacy group in support of preserving biological families. The mission of SOS is:

SOS supports all members of expectant families considering adoption. We are committed to helping them make fully informed decisions based on information that so many other families have learned too late. We are dedicated to ensuring that they avoid applying a permanent solution to a temporary crisis based on partial or misinformation.

SOS is dedicated to direct action and education regarding the preservation of biological families whenever possible. This may include assisting expectant and new parents by locating resources, explaining the long and short term effects of adoption separation on everyone in the natural family, explaining the lifelong effects of trauma their infant will suffer if exposed to maternal separation, and connecting them with a local support person and mentor.

SOS welcomes volunteers, donations and donors to join us in empowering and preserving families by preventing unnecessary adoptions and advocating for fair and ethical adoption laws, policies and practices.

If you would like to support SOS in their work to keep biological families together, please visit their website at www.savingoursistersadoption.org

Womb Writings By Susie Stricker

Profoundly moved by a prompt given for a writing exercise while participating in Flourish, I created a visual for the essay I wrote. The prompt was to imagine I had the ability to communicate to my first mother by writing on the inside surface of her womb. I was asked to consider what I would write if I knew her plans to relinquish me once I was born. The piece expresses how I don't agree with the advice she is getting and staying together is the best thing for both of us. A child should never be taken away from their mother. Period.

I Know This Much Is True By April Gaulke/ Francine J Bauer

This art was inspired by the year I spent in Flourish. Each word consists of letters individually cut from a dictionary page. Within each letter are words describing how this time has influenced me and how adoption has impacted my life. The writing from prompts, conversations and relationships that have evolved from this time have had a powerful effect on my life. While it's impossible to fully understand the impact of being adopted to those who have been fortunate to be raised by first families, I hope this may give some insight into our truth.

Mirroring by Michelle Madsen Hinton

I wanted to convey the duality of being an adoptee in my art piece. I drew orchids; delicate, unique, and extremely fragile. The stems are strong and will grow tall, with support. The roots of some orchids are fully exposed, aerial, not rooted in soil, and will grow on their host. Orchid flowers are mirrored halves. One side mirrors the other.

As adoptees, we too will grow with support, in relation to other adoptees. We don't grow in the soil, but can thrive. Being adopted can feel as though you are two people in one, one that everyone wants you to be, and you.

There are two sections in this piece, top and bottom. On the bottom half, the orchid is surrounded by a murkiness of flower shapes and words from my journal during Flourish: "Rejection leads to terror", "Broken down", "My authentic self was rejected", "What do we risk and for what reward?" With minimal color, I attempt to convey my feelings that I need to remain plain, unseen, always blend in, conforming to a norm to be in relation to the world.

The top half of the piece is how I feel after being in community with other adoptees, the orchid has gained colors, strength, and dare I say confidence. I can be my bright and shiny self, and speak my truths, share hard emotions, grow, all without having to explain why it is such a triumph. The roots are exposed and cut off, yet we survive.

I chose to collage the orchids with layers of rice paper printed with my own adoption court paperwork. The words in the papers are so hard to read as an adoptee; terminate, illegitimate, baby girl, filed.

To show the difficult duality is within adoptees, I sewed the pieces together.

To view the piece as its whole, you see the mirroring. As adoptees we are able to mirror each other through our knowing the lived experience. We validate each other, our feelings, our sorrows, our grief, and our celebrations.

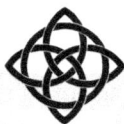

ANN MIKESKA

VIRGINIA

The Year of Flourish

SPENDING ONE DAY A WEEK for an entire year with twenty five adoptees, in a group facilitated by two well-known adoptees – one a writer, one a therapist – sounded amazing, terrifying, and more than a little radical. Always one to suffer from both extreme procrastination and Fear of Missing Out (FOMO) I eventually signed up and as luck would have it, got the very last spot. I was both unprepared and naive to the enormous impact such a group would have on me.

We in Flourish are spread out across the USA and globe. We are diverse in education, career field, lifestyle, family composition, income bracket, and age. Yet, at our very core, where it matters most, we are strikingly similar. We love, we hurt, we long for acceptance and connection. Before we were anything we were the unwanted, the ones not kept, born in shame and secrecy, relinquished, illegitimate, we were bastards.

Each week the fortresses of high walls constructed over decades of self-preservation developed cracks; we afforded our fellow Flourishers peeks at feelings long held close if not kept in total silence. Over the months the cracks turned into openings, windows into our souls, doors of acceptance. Watching the faces of 25 people mirroring my feelings, nodding in agreement and understanding in unison, and simply getting "it" without a word of explanation is an ineffable feeling. It often felt like we were connected with an invisible string, tightly woven into one unified being.

Pam and Anne wanted to create something exceptional, grassroots, to duplicate and curate friendships like their own among other adopted people. The idea for Flourish was born out of this desire. Not only did they succeed, we flourished, we evolved and bloomed into something no one could have imagined a year ago. Pam and Anne formed a group and gently eased it along until it picked up speed, grew large and powerful, and we became a force unto ourselves. The year was an intangible gift full of validation and belonging.

The twelve months were not without conflict or disagreements; there were misunderstandings, feelings were hurt, tears were shed. No group experience, even with the best of outcomes, is ever without growing pains and occasional friction. In the end, I believe we are one cohesive group, sharing an unbreakable bond. Over the year, I've realized the importance of community, of acceptance, of non-judgement, validation, kindness, and trust. I know I am not alone; I will never be alone. I would walk through the pits of Hell for every single one of these spectacular human beings. I trust they would do the same for me.

My wish for all adoptees is to find your people. Read books written by adoptees, listen to adoptee-produced podcasts, join Facebook pages and support groups. We all long for connection and acceptance. Not only is connection an antidote to loneliness, being surrounded by people who reflect your feelings, who meet you where you are, who hold space and sit with you in both pain and happiness is incredibly healing. We all deserve to feel loved.

Womb Writing: Words to my First Mother

We shared a life, you and I, physically connected in the way only a mother and her child can be. I knew the sound of your voice, the tempo of your heartbeat, the gait of your walk. The rhythm of you lulled me to sleep, caressed me in warmth and security. I didn't know how soon it would end, how quickly I would be all alone, permanently severed from not only you and the rest of our family, and from the me I was supposed to become.

I'm left with shadowed memories, longing for what should have been, missing someone I can't remember. I cried myself to sleep hundreds of nights during my childhood because the grief and ache of a loss I couldn't name or understand never dulled. It was constant in my life. I was four years old the first time I wanted to die. The pain was unbearable. I wanted it to end.

I was always searching. Searching faces in crowds, on TV, every passerby on the street. Looking for familiar eyes, a spark of recognition, something, anything. I needed to fill the emptiness, the ever-present void. When you left my newborn baby-self alone in the hospital you didn't see my gaping wound, you didn't hear my primal scream. Perhaps you will listen now.

If I could turn back time to before I was born, knowing what I know now, I would leave my handprints on the wall of your womb, proof that I was there, proof that I existed. I'd write an infinite number of words on your womb. I would write a novel for those who will later be cocooned within these same sacred walls to read as they too enjoy the safety of your body. The children you kept, nurtured, and loved – my siblings. I would leave pieces of my story for them to find and carry to you. I would not allow my existence to be a secret. They would leave your body with the knowledge of me.

The story I would tell you is one of infinite loss. I would beg you not to listen to your mother. Do not listen to the social workers at the home where you were sent. You won't forget you had a baby and move on with your life. They are liars. I would implore you to fight with every ounce of mental and physical strength you possess to keep me. Please do not make a permanent decision for what will be an extremely temporary situation. It will be alright; we will be alright together. My dad will make it out of the war alive. He will return to you. He loves you. You love him. You will marry and the two of you will cherish each other for decades. You will go on to have other children with him and still feel the loss you were never allowed to grieve. The loss will impact you in a multitude of ways. You will suffer in silence. The ghost of your lost baby will follow you throughout your life. Please don't let me become a ghost.

My story will tell how our separation from each other and the loss of you has had an impact on my life, and how the abandonment I was born into has woven its way into my very core. I've always felt unmoored, floating in nothingness. I became a chameleon, flawlessly changing into what people wanted me to be. Never knowing who I truly am. Never trusting I was good enough. These thoughts have been entwined with every relationship I've had. My marriage has been strained at times by my unrealized trauma. My children suffered because I unknowingly would not allow myself to fully attach to them. They reached for me, and I stepped back. My soul mourns for what they lost, for the mother they deserved. For the mother I didn't know how to be.

Mommy, please do not leave me. I need you. I have always needed you. I have always missed you.

Please don't become a ghost.

Adoption

Being an adopted person is complicated. It's layers upon layers of paradoxes. It's duality. It's *and* and *both*. At times it's beyond comprehension let alone explanations.

As a child I often heard common phrases about adoption: "You were chosen." "Your mother loved you so much but couldn't afford to take care of you so gave you to someone who could." "We prayed for a baby and God gave us you." "You were given a better life." "You must be so grateful your parents adopted you." "Aren't you glad your real mom didn't have an abortion?" Although well-intended, these phrases caused immeasurable damage.

Knowing I was chosen, I'd always pictured a room full of bassinets neatly lined up in rows, each containing a baby awaiting a family. I had imagined my parents walking from baby to baby, gazing at each, wanting to pick the very best one, and realizing upon seeing me, I was the perfect daughter for them. At age nine or 10, cuddled up on the couch reading next to my mom, my head comfortably resting upon her breast, I looked up at her and asked how many babies they had to choose from before deciding on me. She gave me a quizzical look and said, "Just you. You were the baby we had waited and prayed for." My world collapsed. I can still feel the heaviness of my body. In that moment, I realized they didn't *choose* me; they took the only baby offered. They would have happily taken and loved any baby given to them just as much as they loved me. I could have easily been given to a different couple. What would have happened if I went home with another family? I would have a different name, a different life, another mom and dad. I felt the randomness of adoption in my soul. That was the last day I ever cuddled with my mom.

The axis of my world shifted that day. I internally questioned everything I'd been told and believed about adoption. Every well-intended claim about adoption now had a very different meaning; darker and more sinister.

For reasons I was unaware of at the time, my adoptive family had struggled financially for many years. I'd heard the "She loved you so much she gave you to someone who could take better care of you" countless times. I knew my parents loved my brother and I very much. I also knew they didn't have enough money to pay the bills many months. Were they going to give us away to a family who could better afford to take care of us? Isn't that what parents who love their children do? I was terrified I'd come home from school and a rich family would be there waiting to make me their daughter, hoping they would also want my younger brother. Could we be separated?

I questioned God. Why would He choose to make my mom unable to carry a baby and instead put me in someone's body who wasn't able to take care of me? Wouldn't it have been better for everyone to just put me in the right mommy? Did my parents really pray for someone to not be able to raise their own child so they could have it instead? To my child-mind, that seemed very unkind and cruel.

I hated being adopted. What I wanted was to be my parent's biological daughter. I wanted to look like my family. I wanted to hear people say things like "Oh, you get your eyes from your mom, or you inherited grandma's laugh." I was never grateful to be adopted and I knew I was supposed to be.

Since being in reunion with my family of origin I've realized everything I missed by not growing up with them. They are truly my people and I love them beyond words. We share blood, we share ancestors, we share many commonalities, yet we don't share a history, we don't share memories. We missed decades together that we can't recapture. The magnitude of loss is unfathomable. Adoption guarantees a different life, not a better life.

Adoption for me has meant loving two families and truly belonging to neither.

ANN'S STORY:

I am a "Baby Scoop Era" adoptee. I was relinquished at three days old, placed in some type of foster care/baby home for several weeks, and eventually placed with my adoptive parents at 10 weeks old. They were my guardians until my adoption was finalized when I was 14 months old. I was raised with a younger, also adopted, not biological brother. My adoptive name was Ann. I learned upon reunion my name at birth was Heather. My husband and I had serendipitously named our eldest daughter Heather. I've known I was adopted for as long as I can remember. It's always been a part of my story. My adoptive parents both passed away many years ago. My adoptive brother and I have an ongoing sibling relationship. I have been in reunion with my entire first family for almost four years. I was 50 years old when I found them. My first parents married when I was five months old and I have two full biological siblings. My sister, who is my very best friend, is two and a half years younger than me and my brother is five and a half years younger. I also have three older half siblings from my dad's first marriage.

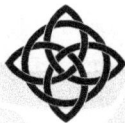

CATIE SAMANTHA PECK

NEW YORK

Spring Onions

SOMETIMES REFERRED TO AS SCALLIONS or green onions, this vegetable is an onion that is harvested before maturity is reached.

These onions have a root end that you often trim off before using the green stalks in recipes.

After the onions are diced and used for their culinary destiny, the unrooted bulb is most often discarded; given to waste or compost.

Consider that you can place a used up, unrooted bulb ('scrap') in a container of water with other bulbs.

They are not garbage because they have been used, they are unplanted and feel small.

You can encourage those root ends to grow!

Once their roots are in a container with enough water with others they will grow tall. Strong.

They will not be rooted in soil like most other plants. They're floating in water, not growing in the ground where they were originally planted! Madness!

They often grow quickly.

Lush, green beauty.

They're zesty.

They grow: Even though they are not rooted.

If you don't cut the greens down over time, the plant could get to be much larger than the green onions you find in your grocery store!

Walking through the kitchen one spring day, my husband remarked, "You are the green onion growing in the jar."

Uprooted due to my relinquishment at birth, yet growing amongst other uprooted people, finding my voice, finding my biological family, finding myself.

GROWING without planted roots.

Spring onions.

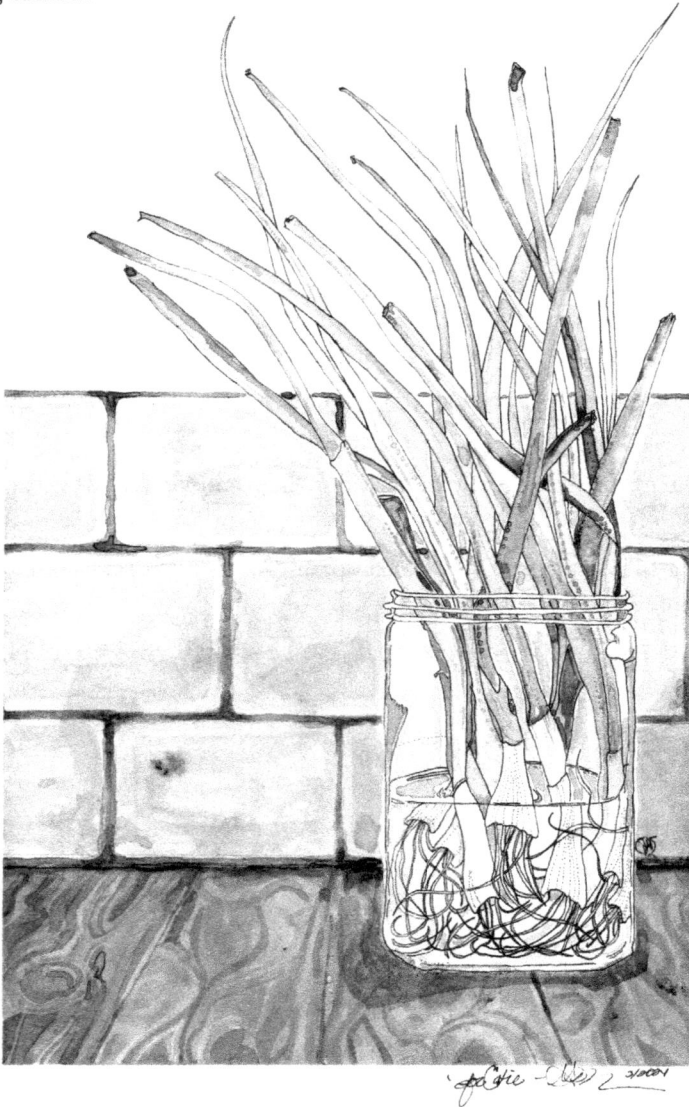

Artist **MICHELLE HINTON**

Flourish, a poem

Born and at once-alone!

Placed under gaslight for warmth.

The clink of coins for a lullaby.

Belonging only to self now.

Chameleon for others.

Adopt/adapt.

Lost.

Untethered.

Seeking.

A family of friends forged in courage and voice.

There. Are. Others.

Together, We Rise!

The Year of Self Trust

When I really sit with it, and look at it for a long while, I realize that the magnitude of what we lose, as adopted people, is incalculable. The grief is so utterly enormous and so permeated into all that we become from the point of our relinquishment on that those that were kept truly can't understand it. And those of us that weren't kept can hardly untangle it all or language it for you. It is an entirely different way of existing. It's a person who has been at least two people. In one. It's a life experience that the world just can't fully grasp.

Our voices are getting louder in the 2020's. Community is integral. Through community we learn that the thoughts that we have been living with all of our lives, and that we have developed very specific coping strategies to manage, are not only common, but a normal reaction to an abnormal situation. These strategies are needed to exist in the world with non-adopted people. It's not

Normal to grow up in a family you are not genetically related to with no access to your biological history.

In the desolate Silo of "I don't belong here...where are my real parents?" it can be hard to do the simple stuff like picking what cereal to eat for breakfast, much less explain your complicated feelings about not knowing where your first family is or why you don't know what your ethnicity is. In a community of true belonging and authentic self and authentic voice, suddenly the truth of the matter just pours out ....drip drip drip drip drip ... GUSH.

Through my year of Flourishing in an adoptee community, I developed an unwavering ability to trust myself.

My experiences ... are not so big and isolating and terrifying anymore.

Through the mirroring and attunement of other adoptees my growth was propelled.

I found my agency. The antidote to trauma.

My inner voice, once shuttered, shaved off, marginalized, shapeshifted for adoption now SCREAMED!

Like a call and response, I'd send out the need for emotional help or understanding to other adoptees and they'd come. At various states in their own adoption journey there they were with their container, ready.

Waiting. Fill my bowl. I can take it. Let it out. Here are my hands ... pour your thoughts onto them. Cry your tears. I am your people. My mother left me too. GUSH.

Trusting Myself in the Year of Flourish: Evidence.

- I ordered my original birth documents, I trusted I could live through what they said. I trusted I was ready for whatever they would reveal to me. I opened them.

- I contacted a search angel, I trusted I could live through what she found even though it would change all the things I knew about myself to be true. I took her call.

- I went away alone to a cabin in the woods to process this. I trusted I was ready to hold all of this by myself. Not only ready but I NEEDED to hold this by myself. My only companion – nature. It can hold the enormity of this grief. I came home.

- I wrote letters to my first family – my biological Mom and my biological Dad – and I trusted that I could hold and sustain and endure whatever the outcome was. I mailed them.

- Summer Solstice. The longest days of the year. The week of my 37th birthday. I picked up the phone when both parents called and I trusted I could tolerate whatever they said and whatever I learned about me. I kept picking up.

- I asked all the questions I could muster. I laid my big feelings right on the table. We ate dinner alongside them. We tucked them in at night. We danced with our feelings until our feet all hurt. I keep asking.

- I told the truth to my adoptive Dad, I trusted that I could survive however he reacted. He keeps listening. I keep talking.

- I told the truth to my first parents. All the truth. They keep listening. I keep talking.

- I trusted my marriage. I was expanding. He was sharing me now. There was no going back. He keeps choosing me. All versions.

- I trusted those closest to me would stick around. I wasn't around for a long while. You might see my body but my mind was out to sea. Bobbing among the waves. So far from shore. Trying on different lives in my mental ocean while you eat your tuna sandwich. My quest was my purpose now. They still love me.

- I met my birth mother. Her. HER. I met my birth mother. I trusted I was ready and I wanted that relationship in my life. The shift in my body was cellular. Her heartbeat is Home. I kept meeting her.

- I met my birth father, I trusted I was ready and I wanted that relationship in my life. We mutually adore and respect each other. He didn't know. He didn't know he created a whole person. I kept meeting him.

- I met my half siblings, I trusted I was ready and I wanted those relationships in my life. They're wonderful people! Imagine what they had to consider, accept, reckon with about their father? Their concept of family? And they showed up for me. We're gonna keep going.

- I met some extended maternal and paternal family trusting I was ready and I wanted those relationships in my life. That journey is only beginning. We're gonna keep going.

- I trusted that my life purpose was shifting. That I would take my social work career and instead of serving veterans, I would serve adopted people. This is my calling. My voice is needed. I can help others. I must. I know my purpose.

- I trusted that a book was coming from my heart out through my fingertips. I prioritized writing. The middle of the night. In airports. On airplanes. On breaks at work. In a Kansas cemetery. On Lake Michigan. In the car with my husband driving to Maryland. By the pool at an Orlando resort. Looking at the Pacific Ocean. In the Blue Ridge Mountains. On a balcony in Annapolis. Keep writing.

I trusted myself over and over and over again this year and I was right. I kept moving towards my true north and my best interests each and every time. It was terrifying. It was exceptionally worth it. It was gutting. It was exhilarating. It was heartbreaking. It is a gorgeous adventure. I am just getting started.

CATIE'S STORY:

I was relinquished at birth, placed in 2 foster homes, then adopted at 7 weeks old through LDS Family Services (the Mormon church). My first mother was 17 years old at the time of my birth and wished to keep her baby. Due to church doctrine that shamed instead of supporting unmarried, pregnant women and lack of support from her family she felt she was without choices. This trauma impacted the rest of her life and she never had other children. I was raised as an only child. I do not have a memory of when I learned I was adopted; it feels like I always knew that fact. My name at birth was Samantha Claire and was changed at the time of my adoption to Catherine Anne. I am changing my name to Catie Samantha to reflect and reclaim my original name. Searching at age 36, I am now in a successful reunion with both parents and maintain relationships with my first mother, first father, and my two paternal half siblings; I have also positively connected with many other extended biological family members. My adoptive family is supportive of my journey and I am in relationship with all of my living parents at this time.

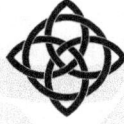

CHRISTINE FUHRMAN-CAMERON

KANSAS

One Year In Flourish

I'M AN ADOPTEE. I'm also a therapist who initially read *The Primal Wound: Understanding the Adopted Child*, by Nancy Verrier (1993), twice – once as an undergraduate and again in graduate school. I somehow managed to be so disconnected from my own truth that it didn't even dawn on me that this book applied to me in any shape or form. It should be noted that the professional mentors I had around me often reinforced the idea that infant adoption is beautiful and not even remotely noteworthy from a clinical perspective. Fast forward 14 years into a career working with kids in foster care and young people who aged out of the system. Keep going into 20 years of reunion with my maternal family and 7 years past secondary rejection with my bio father. Add on three more years to the part where I'd find out I have another biological brother. I finally read *The Primal Wound* a third time and just about died.

My brain became flooded with a slow motion movie screen highlighting memories of information - doled out by my adoptive parents, the Catholic Church I was raised in and society throughout the years. I was sold to my parents for $10,000 under the false belief that they were buying a blank slate. My parents were praised throughout my life for saving me and often would remind me too. Despite the blank slate storyline, there were comments about how my biological mother was a promiscuous teen who got caught up with a deadbeat, older guy. My childhood brain stored this information as evidence to support the belief that I am bad.

I came with a one page, one-sided piece of paper. It was non-identifying and composed of two columns, one for the birthmother and maternal grandparents and the other for the birthfather and paternal grandparents. This document contained demographics in each column – height, weight, hair color, eye color, bone structure, overall health status, and religious affiliation. The document was so formal and although the typed letters filled one full page, it couldn't have been more vague. If you read it too quickly, you'd likely miss the personal characteristics that were listed for each respective birthparent. To me, these typed words were more valuable than my Mattel Dance Club Barbie who came with her own cassette tape. It said my birthmother was "vivacious, energetic, sense of humor, likable, good student" while my birthfather was reportedly "soft-spoken, easygoing, sensitive, good student." These little nuggets of gold provided a loose tangible connection to where I came from. Yet the way in which it was typed up felt dismissive, as if it wasn't real, I wasn't real. No photographs. No names. Perhaps where I came from was so immoral that these little tidbits of information were all that was left to share. The one piece of information that wasn't on this document but that was acceptable enough to be talked about as part of me in this new family was my Italian heritage. It also made me stand out against my fair skinned, Irish adopted brother who was mirrored in complexion by our Irish Catholic adoptive parents. Since I can remember, I searched everywhere; eyes, hands, face, hair, smile, anything that looked like it could be a part of me. The reality that I read *The Primal Wound* three times before it finally knocked me on my ass is actually not that hard to believe at all.

In my late 30's, following my third reading of *The Primal Wound*, I became desperate to find people like me … adoptees. I joined every adoptee-related Facebook group but nothing ever resonated. It took more than a year of searching for some kind of understanding before my partner finally talked me into looking for a podcast. She'd heard enough of my ranting that I can't focus anytime I'd tried podcasts before. Despite my stubbornness, I chose to scroll through Apple podcasts the next morning while sitting in my car. I stumbled upon a show titled *Adoptees On*, hosted by adoptee Haley Radke. "Adoptees," I said to myself. My body felt warm. It was a term I'd never heard before and something about this new word in my vocabulary was like a shock to my system in a way I'll never forget. I fastened my seatbelt and out of the driveway I went. I was on my way to work and had no idea that the universe was about to explode. I wasn't even five miles from home before I had to pull off the highway and onto a side road. I hadn't even listened to a full 10 minutes of an episode I had randomly pressed "play" on but I was about to become immobilized. The two guests were adoptees, one a writer and the other was a therapist. An adopted therapist, like me. My brain thought it was misfiring. Tears were rolling down my cheeks, onto my freshly laundered sweater. It was as if the floodgates I'd worked so hard to maintain literally came crashing down with such force I couldn't have stopped them if I tried. What had felt like a dirty secret I had hidden so deeply inside of me was beginning to emerge with a force I couldn't delay. These women were speaking a new language with such compassion and confidence. Every cell in my body was tingling as if I were being brought to life for the first time. Either that or I was having a flashback of the summer I spent consuming magic mushrooms while camping with friends. I was hungry to learn this new language that resonated inside of me as it was providing an explanation to the jumble of emotions and duality I've felt since day one. Needless to say, I didn't go to work that day.

Following a year of listening to every episode of *Adoptees On* (many repeatedly) along with attending an adoptee conference and retreat, I was starving for more. Connection. I'd already had a taste of what it was like to be in a room full of adoptees after attending a retreat in Berkeley, California hosted by Pam Cordano, MFT and Anne Heffron. It was magical and gut-wrenching all at the same time. The truth was that despite this retreat bringing me a sense of grounding internally, it was incredibly painful when I returned back to the "real world." Best friends I've had for years felt like strangers. I was even further dissociated when around my adoptive family. I didn't know how to communicate with my birth family anymore. My colleagues at work who deemed themselves "attachment specialists" were creeping into the validation and sense of self I'd begun to experience. Society as a whole had 40 years of shoving the whitewashed narrative around adoption down my throat to the point that it was beyond impossible to attempt to unlearn this in the matter of a four-day retreat.

Now trying to sum up the trepidation beforehand and even begin to explain what this year-long experience was like, I have to reflect on the thoughts and feelings I had as I considered taking this plunge into Flourish. Have you ever read or heard about one of those stories where someone trains or dedicates themselves to reaching a goal such as running a marathon, sobriety, climbing Mount Everest, hiking the Appalachian Trail, going on a year-long sabbatical? I love stories like these because they allow me to escape from the belief that I wasn't capable, let alone deserving of an experience so rewarding. My own insecurities made me think that there was no possible way I could indulge in Flourish, a year-long commitment just for my own personal experience of growth, healing and connection. I'm not deserving of something so potentially powerful.

Many people around the world were already isolated due to the pandemic. I was longing for more as I was post two years from the adoptee retreat and still trying to find my way, to feel a sense of being rooted. I'd tasted this for four days while in Berkeley so a part of me knew it was possible. While the weekly sessions with my non-adoptee therapist were helpful in many ways, having to over-explain myself, provide disclaimers and educate her on adoptee trauma only fed into the issues I was there for in the first place.

The commitment to attend this group every week for two hours for a solid 12 months tapped into the insecurities and fear inside my infant self. My default network wanted to take over taunting me with the thoughts that I'd be an outsider, nobody would like me, whatever I'd say would be stupid, I won't fit in. I'm definitely not a writer. I'm not enough. It's selfish to take up this much time simply because of my experience as an adoptee. The relinquished baby inside of me wanted to scream and flail and the adult in me wanted to hold her and push through the discomfort. I sent a frantic email to Anne and Pam asking for written assurances that an emergency exit was available. They reassured me and encouraged me to commit for one month and see how it goes. I can do this. That's not that big of a deal, right?

The first Zoom class on a cold day in January 2021 was initially terrifying. It brought me back to growing up in my adopted family and sitting at the dinner table where I quickly learned to conceal all parts of myself that were deemed different, unacceptable or even "ridiculous." My body was painfully rigid. Trying to regulate my breathing was a battle, as if I was 50 feet below sea level with cinder blocks tied to my limbs. And at the same time I looked across the screen at the faces of adoptees from multiple countries, ages, races, ethnicities, and genders. A part of me couldn't help but feel like this was going to be an experience that was going to kick my ass in the best way possible. My spine felt tickles and the goosebumps rose to the surface. We all made a choice to be here, as adoptees.

And then came our first writing prompt: *Who are you in a nutshell?* We were asked to write without disclaimers or softening parts of self in order to make it more palatable for others. My mind went blank. I don't even know who the fuck I am. I've spent four decades of my life molding into whomever I thought others wanted me to be at the time. It was enough to send my nervous system into a full blown panic attack.

As we finished writing I heard Anne's voice saying something about how we'd go around the room and share what we wrote. Pam chimed in with a polite statement about how it was voluntary but my brain and body didn't absorb it as such. I'm pretty sure I was levitating at this point. I'm not a writer. I don't even remember what I wrote but I was certain it wouldn't be accepted. Holy shit how do I get out of this? I could pretend I'm having Wi-Fi issues and just bail. Before I knew it, the first person started reading what she had written. I became completely entranced. Tears rolled down my face. I didn't even bother to wipe them away. My body was warm again. The words she and others read aloud that day and every single week in Flourish mirrored all that I had locked in a secret compartment deep beneath the surface and buried in shame. What kept coming to mind was some quote I'd read by Maggie Kuhn, "Speak your mind even if your voice shakes." I chose to lean in, to take the risk. Be vulnerable.

There's something unbelievably motivating about knowing this was voluntary and seeing a Zoom room full of adopted people who shared the feelings and thoughts and hopes and grief I'd kept inside of myself. It was equally powerful to the first time I laid eyes on my birthmother when I was 18. For the first time in my life, I saw myself reflected in another human being. And here again at 40, something similar was happening in the moment that would take more than a year to name.

This year-long direct experience in Flourish made me feel real. I am a real live human being. I am understood. I am not alone. I am seen, even in silence. More than anything, I am safe. Flourish became a space where there's no need for disclaimers about gratitude in order to protect others in the adoption constellation or appear ungrateful. This experience gave validation and meaning to the suffering. It began to fill in the gaps of not knowing or understanding. I had found my tribe, a place of belonging.

Twelve months later, I'm not sure if I can say it ever got easier to read aloud what I'd written but what I can say without any doubt is that with each and every Flourish class, I got closer to my truth and myself. I began to find my authentic voice. I reflect on that first writing prompt about who I am in a nutshell and now I can provide answers from my heart. I began to learn what it is like to move energy away from the fawning response of trauma and into your body. Do you know how unbelievably liberating it is to know definitively just exactly what it feels like in your body when you are speaking your truth? It is a newfound freedom and comfort I imagine must be somewhere close to the experience of an unborn child safely in its mother's womb. I can now say with certainty that I am a sensitive soul who feels deeply. I am a passionate lover. I thrive on being independent yet find comfort in a helping hand. I love to feel dirt on my feet and hands. The sights and sounds of bodies of water regulates my breathing faster than any yoga class I've attended. Climbing mountains makes me feel like a badass warrior. Being in nature is where I feel the safest. I came out of the womb a helper and a healer. I am soft and strong and stubborn. What emerged from within me was a voice speaking truth without the bullshit layer on top. A voice I didn't know I had but longed for. A voice that might shake but is full of strength. Validation. Purpose. I am rooted and now I Flourish.

My Place at the Table

DISCLAIMER: The following includes information pertaining to suicide and may be triggering or difficult for readers.

In the center of the hearth room that opens up into the kitchen was a large, oval table made of thick, sturdy walnut. The wood stain highlighted its natural grain as if it were a work of art. It was always covered with a tablecloth that changed with seasons while the centerpieces rotated in and out as the holidays came and went.

The effort my adoptive parents went to in order to protect this table's pristine finish wouldn't make sense to me until decades later. The table became symbolic and disorienting. How could they be aware of the care that was required for this table to last and remain beautiful and sturdy but were completely oblivious to the attention and care I needed to become and feel beautiful and sturdy? Confident in myself and who I was. I was a "blank slate" so why would I require such effort?

While I found this table beautiful, my experiences seated here were not.

We had assigned seats. I sat next to my older, also adopted brother while our parents sat across from us. On occasion my dad would take his place at the head of the table, especially if we had guests. Blue plate for my brother, pink for me and yellow or green for the parents. We even had matching bowls and cups. I'll admit there was a part of me that did feel special having my own pink colored plate despite this inner knowing that I was sitting at a table not meant for me.

I watched TV shows and movies almost in envy when family dinner table scenes would come on. I often wondered why the table I sat at never mirrored the family disputes, emotional outbursts, deep talks or genuine laughter over inside jokes I saw on the screen. Hollywood, along with meals shared with friends and other families, tricked me into believing that all these tables were meant for coming together. A place for genuine family connection, a place to feel safe and secure sharing thoughts and feelings, the good, the bad and everything in between with acceptance and acknowledgement. A place for being real.

I learned relatively quickly that this wasn't like the other tables I had seen or sat at. This table was more like a grand inquisition into my life filled with judgment. It wasn't about safety or acceptance, it was all about expectations. And the expectations at this table were quite different. I was routinely asked a series of questions about the status of my chores, homework, grades, friendships, sports, and other activities. How I needed to look and behave were went over like a checklist of what I had to do in order to be "loved and accepted" at this "table" and in this family unit. The message was clear: I need to look and behave in such a way that reinforced the perception that my parents were good parents and I was grateful to have been saved.

Shame is all this table fed me throughout my younger years. It taught me to make myself smaller. It gave me years of experience stifling my intuition and self-worth. It muted my creativity as it demanded that I not color outside the lines. It silenced my voice and shut down my opinions if they differed from those seated around me. Any expression of emotion that created discomfort for the adults seated here was unacceptable. This reinforcement tightened my throat in ways that will take a lifetime to unwind. In turn, there was no conversation about these emotions or feelings. I was treated like the odd one out and looked it too.

I became numb.

This table rewarded compliance, perfectionism and a layer of bullshit so as to keep others feeling good about themselves. The seat I occupied and the role in which I was expected to assume at this table kept me in the closet for almost 30 years suppressing my queer self.

This table force fed the lies my parents ate up from Catholic Charities that I am a blank slate. I must bury (deeply) the parts of self that are different from those seated at this table if I want to be accepted. Kept.

My time at this table taught me not to take up space and even more so, that I should be forever grateful for taking a seat at it. It led me to believe that where I came from was no good and therefore I am no good.

Despite all of the confusion, the pain, I tried my damnedest to earn a spot at this table.

As I came into my teenage years, the nature within me was relentless and persistent. The longing for any breadcrumb of knowledge about where I came from was in constant conflict with the narrative that I was a blank slate. The reinforcement of demands from those around this table to shut off any parts of me deemed unacceptable was too much for my "overly sensitive" self.

The first time I lost my place at this table was a couple of weeks before my 15th birthday – the same age in which my biological mother became pregnant with me. To be fair, I didn't give my parents' much choice in the matter as I tried to end my life. The madness and overwhelming feelings of hopelessness became too much inside of me. If I was told one more time that I was "chosen" I'm fairly certain my body would have combusted on its own. I never felt chosen. My brain couldn't even compute the notion. These words ricocheted off of my skin as if the core inside my body knew it was utter bullshit. Lies. The very few adults I tried to talk with to gain a compassionate ear only fed me with the same rhetoric. I should be grateful. I am lucky to have been saved and given a "better" life.

What if I didn't want to be saved?

Since nobody asked, I decided to try to take matters into my own hands.

That year was full of several hospitalizations. Puking blue foam after overdosing on pills in an attempt to put a stop to the gut-wrenching disgust I had within myself. Days turned into weeks with monitors attached to my chest due to the irregularities in my broken heart. The weeks turned into months confined within the walls of a residential treatment center where I'd begin accumulating frequent flier miles. Never- ending side effects due to the psychiatrist not being able to find the magic pill that would "fix" me. Hours-long intensive family and individual therapy sessions, which often led to explosive blow-ups between my father and I before I'd run out of the room defeated, unheard and completely unseen. Barely a mention of how my being relinquished or that I'm adopted might all be related. In fact, the only nod to my being adopted came directly from a psychiatrist following one of those family therapy sessions where this woman looked at me and said "It's because you're adopted." This statement solidified what I already knew, I was damaged. Unwanted. Bad.

Back and forth dialogue continued between my parents and therapist about whether or not I should be moved to the group home across the field at Florence Crittenton's Children's Center, formerly known as the Florence Crittenton Home for unwed mothers. Just about every room in the residential units gave way to a view of this group home, almost as if it was a reminder of what happens to kids who don't get "fixed." The group home, called Carrier House, was a catch-all for many like myself who'd been adopted. But living at that place would mean I would be un-adopted.

I begged and pleaded. Promised to be better. Regurgitated lines over and over about being grateful. "Perhaps there are other options," I heard my therapist say as she went on to talk about boarding schools. My parents leaned into her, clearly interested in the possibilities and soaking up her ideas. They were desperate. And it was as if I wasn't even in the room.

I felt ashamed for existing. For being such a burden. For being me. Overcome with guilt for not finishing the job and allowing these people to be free. Free of me.

Back and forth I went, trying to earn a seat at that table.

I'll never forget the fall afternoon of my sophomore year in high school. The apricot colored tablecloth was worn at the edges where I sat due to my unrelenting fidgeting. The cloth hung just low enough in my lap that I could rub the seams relentlessly between my fingers in an effort to soothe the anxiety without anyone having a clue. I kept getting distracted by the primly planted Hawthorn trees on the other side of the patio French doors. I remember feeling a sense of envy as they were evolving with brilliant shades of a bronzed yellow.

Seated at the table with my (adoptive) mother across from me and a woman in the middle who was hired by my parents to send me away for them. A boarding school placement specialist. I don't remember a word of what was said. I do remember my throat being tight and dry. My body stiff while at the same time attempting to look relaxed with excellent posture. A fake yet desperate smile on my face hoping this woman might feel a sense of compassion for me. Maybe she'd think I'm not as bad as they say I am?

I was handed multiple thick folders filled with glossy, staged photos of high-schoolers smiling and engaging with one another as if they weren't shipped off by parents who didn't want them seated at the family table. Descriptions full of absolute bullshit about academic successes, extracurricular activities and parent visiting weekends. All this in an attempt to make me feel a sense of choice in the matter when every single one of us sitting at the table knew the truth.

I pretended to be optimistic and mumbled something about being grateful as I began packing my belongings in preparation for the move to an all-girls Catholic boarding school located in the middle of nowhere Kansas. There was underlying relief in the reality that my parents had options to send me across the country but instead chose somewhere a little over an hour away. Perhaps this meant I was bad, but not bad-bad. Maybe they'd allow for visits home to sit at the table.

I can't quite explain why I even wanted a place at this table. I knew deep down this table fostered such self-hatred and shame yet I wanted a place at it. I wanted to belong somewhere, even if it didn't feel safe, or feel like home.

My Place at the Table Now

Seated at this table as an adult, I have found new meaning and a way in which to unlearn the lessons that fucked me up far beyond the first time I was sent away from this place. Don't get me wrong, there have been years I didn't sit at this table. And times where I have taken a seat only to feel the same flood of shame and desperation in wanting to disappear. There are also times where my physical body will not allow me to take a seat at this table. My nervous system becomes too amped up with the memories my mind wants to forget and instead of sitting down, I find ways to busy myself. I often hear my mom saying "have a seat, relax," and I literally can't, so I don't. There are now meals and visiting that occurs at this table where I make the conscious choice for myself to take a seat. Every single time I choose to sit at this table, I don't just feel like the odd one out, the one who doesn't fit; I know it to be true. I've stopped suppressing what my entire body and mind know to be real. I lean into myself and remind my throat to loosen and my lungs to breathe.

Ironically enough, the same people seated around this table while I was growing up now beg for me to take a seat here. They would love it if I moved back in and sat at this table every single day for the rest of their lives. They are completely unaware of the pain they've caused despite my past attempts to allow them in. I see me, the real me. I no longer need those seated around this table to see who I am. They aren't capable and I am accepting of this. Truth has been one of the most painful and rewarding gifts I have ever come to know. I now have a choice as to whether or not I want to sit down. I don't need approval anymore.

Seated at this table in present time, I am now the glue. I am the softness that balances the hard. I am no longer uncomfortable in knowing what I say or express may cause uneasiness or disagreement. I am a teacher of truth seated at this table. I am the understanding and openness they didn't know how to give. I am the validation they didn't know I needed yet they ask for regularly today. I am the loyalty they don't deserve. Loyal not out of guilt or gratitude. Instead this loyalty comes from the nature within me, the blood running through my veins. It is the result of a generous and loving heart that knows I'd break theirs if I rejected this seat. I have become the acceptance and safety they never gave. I am the one who calms the storms with compassion instead of shame. I can almost guarantee that those seated here with me always leave this table feeling better because I am the heart. I am the love and I know they feel it too.

The people seated around me at this table are the exact same along with the tablecloths and revolving centerpieces. I cannot even count the number of times I've sat at this very table and admired the row of Hawthorns still on display. Mesmerized by the duality of beautiful white flowers peeking through the large, intimidating thorns. These trees are a standing testament to strength and adaptability. Throughout the years these trees have grown stronger, bolder and more beautiful. Like me.

CHRISTINE'S STORY:

I was relinquished when I was eight days old. I spent a few days in a foster home following my birth while my biological mother, who was 16 at the time, dealt with her own uncertainty. It was ultimately her father who made the final decision that I would be relinquished through Catholic Charities. The following day, I was sent to a new home with a couple who would become my adoptive parents a year later. They already had a two year old son, who was also adopted through Catholic Charities. My birth parents named me Chasity Marie, which was then voided by the state of Kansas and changed by my adoptive parents to Christine Elizabeth. I am still on the journey of reclaiming myself. I never remember not being adopted, it was something told to me at an early age. My adopted brother and I were given a children's book explaining adoption although it never quite aligned with how I felt inside. I longed for my birth mother throughout those years. On my 18th birthday I went to Catholic Charities and a few days later was reconnected with my birth mother and younger, full biological brother. I've been in reunion with my entire maternal family for a little more than over 20 years. I experienced secondary rejection from my biological father in 2007. In 2019 we reconnected and are still in reunion today.

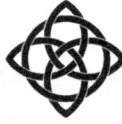

COLEEN NEVIN

THE BRONX

Awaken, Acknowledge, Grow and Flourish

I WAS RAISED AS THE MIDDLE CHILD in a family of three siblings and adopted through Catholic Charities in NYC. I grew up in a large extended Irish-American family. My adoptive parents cared for us and provided us with a family and a loving, safe home. As any young couple would, they had planned for a family that would come naturally. During my journey I have realized and acknowledged that their decision to adopt was rooted in their own grief and loss. There was the loss of their ability to have their own biological children. Adoption was not their first choice no matter how much they loved us. Therefore, the societal narrative that I was chosen was something that permeated my existence and was something that I clung to for many years. The honest reality is that I was not chosen. I was the next baby the Catholic Home Bureau had available. My parents have been deceased for almost 18 and 15 years. I wish I had just one more day to ask them about my first days with them and so much more.

My birth mother found my identity and location when I was an adolescent.

Catholic Charities placed me in a home just a few miles away from her, despite feeding her the fabricated story that I was being placed in a wealthy home in a northern suburb. This was all to add to the falsehood that financial means would give me a "better" life. This was a passive aggressive attempt to intimidate an unwed teenage mother. Our proximity to each other through our lives led the way for years of intertwining and overlapping within our community and within both my birth and adoptive families. These events increased my feelings of being out of control. I went through my teen years with a sense of hypervigilance that grew and was coursing its way through every aspect of my life. I had to ensure that I kept everything in line so that the chaos within me was not something anyone who loved me would see. I had to show that I was all anyone would ever want me to be DESPITE being adopted.

I gave birth to my first child at almost 22 years old. My son was the first person who was biologically connected to me. He was the first person who had my genes, my characteristics, my blood. He was mine and I felt an overwhelming sense of contentment. This feeling made me yearn to enter a reunion with my birth family. I did this with no planning and no support. I wanted to become a part of this perfect family I saw in the photos my birth mother sent to me. My birth mother and birth father reconnected and then shortly after locating me they married. They went on to have two boys who are my biological brothers, 14 and 17 years younger than me. When I reflect on our almost 30-year reunion I see five people brought together by a situation that no one would ever dream of having to go through. My brothers were young children when we met. I would bring them to my home, and they played with my children. My children were closer in age to them than their own biological sister. My brothers would call these two people I just met "mom and dad" so easily. This struck me to the core. This was one example of how I underestimated how reunion would impact me. I did not give myself compassion during this time. I did not allow myself to feel the deep emotions around this. I pushed through always with a smile on my face showing the world again how well I could manage this and make it all perfect too. I also underestimated the impact our reunion would have on my husband and four children. Their love and support for me never failed, but I tried for many years to not even open my emotions to them. I never allowed them to see my inner pain and self- doubt. I was strong and I didn't want even the closest people in my life to think differently.

I believe times of estrangement, absence and preexisting traumas had a profound effect on all of us. These factors have negatively impacted my relationships with my biological family. I have realized years later that I would never truly fit into this immediate family unit. This was no one's fault. How can you attempt to seamlessly become their child or their sibling after a lifetime apart? I have had to forgive myself for feelings of guilt about how my presence or lack of presence in their lives has caused them pain. The times we have spent together were times filled with feelings of joy, sadness, pain, love, shame, connection and detachment. These were also times that I felt the most comfort I have ever felt being in my own skin. I experienced a sense of true belonging. Alternately, there were days I thought I was a stranger in both my adoptive family and in my birth family. It is so completely beyond comprehension for anyone who is not adopted to even imagine what this feels like.

The time spent with my birth mother, birth father and biological siblings and the relationships we have formed have been treasured and valued, yet they have been some of the most challenging times for me. Most days these fractured relationships weigh so heavily on my mind and in my heart. We have attempted to fill in memories and make up for lost time. There has always been an enormous pressure on each of us to be successful with these relationships. This pressure fluctuated between internal and external pressures. Another adoptee described this in a way that fits perfectly. Imagine arriving late to a movie and you are told "don't worry you didn't miss too much – we will fill you in." We are all in pain. We all know we have love for each other. At least in my "adoptee brain" I hope we all have those feelings for each other. We have tried so hard to heal, to accept each other's grief and loss. We are all so deep within our own emotions or disconnected from our emotions that it is challenging to move past the pain into a healthy place of acceptance.

This is the gift of relinquishment and adoption that keeps on giving.

When I reflect on the past 18 months, so many words swirl through my mind and emotions engulf my body. Words like isolation, pain, reckoning, sadness, grief, vulnerability, shame, growth, healing, validation, and truth are at the forefront of many of my thoughts. In September 2020, I began a journey I never knew I needed to take. Since that time, I have slowly begun the process of allowing myself to truly feel the emotions that I have smothered my entire life. I had to give myself permission to prioritize my trauma, my pain, and my grief in a story that I never thought I had the right to say was mine let alone to acknowledge that I needed to heal from. Allowing myself to feel the good and the bad emotions is one of the most challenging things I have had to push myself to do. What I do know is that I would never have survived without the constant presence and lifeline I found within the adoptee community. I have received respect, unconditional love, and a sense of belonging. This community is what has softly held me through this journey. It has supported me and allowed me to find my voice and has helped me to find my true self. This community has enabled me to Flourish.

I was driving home from work one evening that September. I was at the end of almost seven months of working in healthcare during a pandemic, working on a graduate degree in Nursing and had experienced several family losses. 1 felt completely disconnected, sad and lost. I turned on Spotify in the car and decided to try something different. I decided to play an episode of a podcast I had downloaded almost one year before but had never listened to. The podcast was called *Adoptees On*, and the host had a warm and almost familiar voice. I kept listening with cautious anticipation of each word. The voice I came to feel so easily connected to was the host, Haley Radke, also an adoptee. The first episode I listened to was Episode # 3. Haley Radke interviewed an adoptee. I immediately felt at one with this person I had never met. I heard someone else speak the words I would never dare to say. After that first podcast, I absorbed everything adoptee-related that I could find. I had been struggling for the previous year or two with feelings of increasing anxiety, loss of control and an overwhelming heaviness. I read books and listened to other podcasts focused on these very generic issues, but I never felt I was truly getting to the meaning of it all and was only scratching the surface. I assumed that nearing 50, my children getting older and becoming adults and a more stressful job would cause these emotions that I believed were all normal.

After this enlightenment – finally acknowledging this enormous event in my life that I had spent five decades minimizing – I found myself becoming immersed in adoptee books, websites, social media groups, podcasts, and research. I joined an adoptee therapy group among other informal groups. I read psychological studies about the impact of preverbal trauma and Complex PTSD. I read Nancy Verrier's book and learned about the life-long impact of the primal wound when babies are separated from their mothers at birth or shortly after birth. Learning that adoptees are overrepresented in mental health treatment facilities, prisons, and that adoptees are four times more likely than the general population to commit suicide were staggering facts that left me angry and heartbroken for all adoptees. I felt anger towards a society that gaslights the lived experiences of adoptees. I began to process my emotions and create space for the feelings I had buried my entire life. I finally felt a sense of calm when I understood what I was doing was slowly "coming out of the fog." The "coming out of the fog" is a term used to explain the process where adoptees become aware of the reality of adoption and start to integrate the grief, loss and separation surrounding it. I had never heard this term before. This was where my life changed, and I knew I would never be able to go back into the fog.

In my hunger to acknowledge, feel and accept these newfound emotions, I came across several other adoptees who were also guests on *Adoptees On.* They had an impact on me from the moment I heard them speak, especially Pam Cordano and Anne Heffron. They were guests who spoke personally about their experiences as adult adoptees and professionally as a therapist and a writer respectively. I loved listening to their journeys as individuals and as friends. From this friendship grew their idea to form Flourish. The idea was a group of adoptees who would meet weekly via Zoom to write and talk about their lives as adoptees. This idea called to me, yet it frightened me at the same time. It was a one-year commitment to more than 20 adoptees who were strangers. I had no connections to any of them. One year later and this experience has changed my perception of myself as an adoptee and as a human being.

I was born, relinquished, and adopted during the Baby Scoop Era. This was a time when having a baby out of wedlock was looked down upon by society. There was never a consideration for family preservation. There was never a societal advocacy to support the first mother. The normal process was to separate the newborn from the mother and place the newborn in a home with a new family. Adoptive parents were instructed to just raise the child as their own and were not given the tools to support that child through the emotional aspects of their adoption. There was no discussion about the first family the child was removed from. I always knew I was adopted. I don't remember the day or the conversation, but I knew. My story filled the profile of the fairytale adoption story. I fit the family ethnically and even passed for looking like my adoptive family. I was "blessed," I was "chosen" and I was "saved." That was the dialogue the world emphasized. As adoptees our first mothers loved us so much that they sacrificed and gave us away for a better life. This is an incredible burden and weight to carry through life especially when on the inside this was far from how I felt.

I was always the "good adoptee." I don't remember a time in my life that I was not in a state of high alert. I have lived my life never feeling relaxed enough to just breathe and know that I am enough just because I exist. My inner compass was always focused on doing the right thing and never disappointing anyone since I knew deep down in my newborn brain that this might be the reason someone might decide they don't want me, and they choose to leave. This was the pervasive thought that followed me through childhood and into my adult life. Pre-verbal trauma was the impetus for this constant state of intensity and insecurity. I had an inner dialogue of negative self-talk and persistent indecisiveness. I needed to ensure that I did not disappoint. This had an impact on many relationships. It played a part in my roles as a wife, mom, nurse, sister, cousin, friend, daughter.

The role I always played was to adapt like a chameleon. Adoptees have the incredible ability to change and conform to people and situations to fit into a mold that we believe will serve us and assist us to blend in with what the world gives us at the time. We do this with little concern for our own needs or wants. This is most likely a form of self-preservation or protection. It is also a trauma response. Adoptees go from feeling safe and warm within the only protection we knew for nine months into a world of the unknown. Some of us spent months in a state of legal and emotional "limbo." I spent my first six months of life not knowing who cared for me, who I was with or even where I was. The Catholic Church feels it is not important for me to have this information. In a letter from the New York Archdiocese, I was told to be thankful that I was cared for during that time and that they hoped this information would "give me peace to move forward." Those first months in a human's life are the most precious and sacred. Animals are not even taken from their mothers at birth.

I have always looked intently to find behavioral and physical resemblances within families. It fascinated me and then saddened me simultaneously. I yearned for this for my children when I watched them grow and develop relationships with their large paternal family. My husband's family first met me 32 years ago when I visited Ireland for the first time before we were engaged. The physical similarities and characteristics I saw within their family was something so new to me. They had a natural comfort with each other. I feel fortunate to now also call them my family. They have never made me feel different. They never treated me like an outsider despite my own insecurities. As adoptees we live with a lack of genetic mirroring. We look at photos of our adoptive family and their ancestors and realize that these roots and stories are not our own. As I have connected to more biological relatives and distant family, I look at these familiar faces, their characteristics, and I realize this is where I come from and who I am.

When I met my birth mother more than 35 years ago, I did not have the language at that age to comprehend or express the emotions that arose from this huge experience. My adoptive parents and family were limited in their ability to help me navigate through these emotions. Instead, we didn't talk about it. We didn't show emotion or acknowledge the feelings around what was happening. The only conversation I heard happening around me was that my birth mothers' sudden presence in my life had a negative impact on the family. As a teenager, I internalized those words. My very existence was causing pain to so many. I felt guilt and again struggled with an overwhelming sense of wanting to have everything perfect and to not cause any conflict. I have acknowledged that the emotions from that time have been locked deep within me and I have not given myself permission to embrace them. I moved into reunion as a young adult and again never allowed myself to feel. I was married, started my family, began a career and all the while worked to balance the relationships I had developed with my adoptive family and birth family. I spent more than 25 years making sure that everyone else was comfortable. This was no one's fault. I didn't even know that this was what I was doing. I went through our reunion with no professional support, no resources, and with a focus on glorifying this "amazing" story that strangers loved to hear me tell. Even I began to deeply believe the fable of roses, happiness, blessings and being saved. In retrospect, I was pushing myself deeper into the fog the more I told my story and navigated through life. This was until it came crashing in all at once 18 months ago and it forced me to face my truth.

When adoptees speak their truth, they face being labeled as angry adoptees, having mental health issues, ungrateful and damaged. This could not be farther from the truth. Coming out of the fog has given me clarity, self-awareness, self-love, and a greater sense of authentic identity. This is not an identity linked to my biological family, adoptive family or within my own immediate family. It is an acceptance of a true sense of self. I have chosen to be as compassionate to myself as I am to others. I chose a profession based on caring and giving to others. I have spent the past 12 years working in end-of-life care and supporting patients and families through their grief and loss. Through this journey of healing, I am now understanding that something within me pulled me to this work. Having a greater understanding and acceptance of the feelings of loss and grief that will always be with me, helps me to advocate and support those who need it most.

Coming out of the fog and gaining my voice is a daily process. I will always be working to tell myself daily that I am enough. I encourage other adoptees to treat themselves with kindness, and not to apologize for their voice or their truth. No one else has walked in our shoes, no one else knows our heart. We can find strength in community and know that our feelings and our words deserve to be heard.

I want adoptive parents to learn to listen to their child or adult adoptee. Listen and truly hear them. Validate their feelings of curiosity in understanding and possibly knowing their first family. Adoptive parents should not make their adoptive children or adult adoptees feel that they are betraying them for wanting to know who they are. Adoptive parents need to show them acceptance, love, and support when they ask questions. I am only acknowledging so much of my own experience at this point in my life.

I want non-adopted people to just listen. Saying "well, your family loved you and gave you a good life" or "you could have been aborted" or "you were given a better life and should appreciate that" and other statements coming from a place of ignorance and toxic positivity are not supportive.

From my experience within Flourish I can say that I value and have loved my life and the people in it. I have created relationships with my adoptive family that I treasure. They have been with me throughout my life. We have shared memories both joyous and sad that connect us and bond us to each other forever. My life would be different without them in it. I have worked on not allowing my inner thoughts of not truly being a part of my adoptive family to prevail. I am more aware of those who love me unconditionally. They hear me even when I am not saying a word.

Both my immediate and extended birth family have welcomed me and openly expressed "missing" me from the first day they met me. I was always a part of them. I have also built relationships that are so important to me, and I feel very fortunate to even have this opportunity. I know many adoptees who will never have a chance to know and love their birth families. I have made mistakes. I have retracted inside myself with feelings of uncertainty. I have overthought many situations and words said from a place of pain. My fear and insecurities have pushed people away. I am working on not letting those feelings of not being enough creep through any of the relationships I have formed. I am hopeful for continued healing for myself and those I love so deeply. I am hopeful for a sense of acceptance, tolerance, healing, and love for us all.

Adoptees should not have to separate their lives or feel guilty about their emotions or how they feel. We can feel validated that it is OK for us to love the family who raised us and also love our family of origin. Adoptees can have questions and curiosities about where they come from. This does not mean we are betraying our adoptive families. Adoptees can acknowledge that being relinquished and placed for adoption has caused preverbal trauma that has had an impact on our lives. Adoptees are allowed to acknowledge the grief, pain, and loss we feel. We are allowed to heal and speak our truth. We are not blaming our birth family for this. It does not mean that we are blaming our adoptive families for the experience either. It means that WE can love our lives and those in it, but simultaneously allow ourselves to acknowledge our feelings about our story and how it has impacted us.

I look forward to continuing to heal and to traveling on my journey. I look forward to finding continued strength in this community and I hope to participate in advocacy and education around adoption. I look forward to growing in unity with the adoptees who walked this journey out of the fog with me and that I now call my family. We are forever bonded in trust, shared understanding and truth.

I know each one of us will continue to Flourish.

Coleen's Story:

I was born in the Bronx in 1971 in a Catholic Hospital. I was born, relinquished, spent six months in foster care and was then taken home by my adoptive parents and legally adopted almost one year later. This was according to what is written on my adoption agreement and original birth certificate. My birth mom named me Jennifer and gave me her maiden name. She was a 17-year-old girl who did not want to choose relinquishment, but she had no support and not one adult in her life who would listen to her pain. We were both casualties of the transgenerational trauma that she was born into. She had no options and no choice. She experienced this trauma alone. A trauma that would change the course of her life and mine. We would both sadly never be the same.

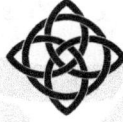

DAWN CONWELL MULKAY

TEXAS

How to Create a Village

"I HAVE BEEN ALONE ALL OF MY LIFE. *Two or more different 'me's' running toward the finish line. I can't get that running time back, but I want to find a way to live in the moment and not even think about the finish line. When I saw this class with Anne and Pam mentioned on Instagram, I thought this might be my only chance to get off the track so I took it. I'm still standing, turning in circles, but I feel my time is here with me.* "

When I joined the Zoom call that first day and saw twenty-five boxes with faces of strangers looking back, I am still surprised I didn't leave. The premise of the class was to meet once a week, have a topic for the month to concentrate on and write about, read our writings out loud to the class and Anne and Pam would be our facilitators.

This may sound like a normal writing class and maybe it was. For this grown-up adoptee, it was terrifying and life-changing. I have never felt comfortable around other people. Growing up, most people didn't understand what I had to say, my perspective, my reasoning. It felt like my total existence was a mystery even to the people who were closest to me; but, to be in an on-line chat room with twenty-five other adoptees was so comforting and validating. It was as if I was pulled from the waters of the Atlantic Ocean, wrapped in a well-used quilt and tucked into an old chair before a roaring fire with hot chocolate, water, chocolate-covered strawberries and my favorite cat napping on my lap.

That first class, Anne and Pam introduced themselves. They talked a bit about the podcast, *Adoptees On*, which is how I became familiar with them both. They outlined the goals for the class, how they meant it to flow and be a living structure which we would create together. They said they weren't there as teacher and therapist, but as companions on the journey. They also talked about the responsibility of being the leaders and organizers of the group and the expectation that we would be responsible members. That we were expected to feel joy, anger, hurt, enthusiasm, otherness, distance, and a myriad of other things and we were expected to share those thoughts and feelings; not bottle them up. This was our first challenge in becoming real. We had to believe that our thoughts and feelings were worthy of being shared and that others might benefit from our sharing.

We wrote about how we felt during class. No explanation, no disclaimers, just read. The amazing thing was no one had to explain what they meant even though we seemed to feel like we should. I know I was so used to explaining, it was difficult to read. In the end, I unmuted myself when I was called on, took a deep breath and read my words aloud, no edits, muted myself and listened to the next person. I did not give myself time to self-criticize. The readings were funny, loving, self-deprecating, heartbreaking and we all understood each other, in the same way that weavers understand the sounds of the fibers as the shuttle passes through or the fishermen understand the anxiety and hope of the next catch. Reading out loud, for someone who spends her time being small, quiet, and as invisible as possible, is terrifying. I read these words that first day:

"I feel like I've been heard. Like I have a right to ask if you've heard me, if you are here with me. I feel like I can start to recognize when I am walking out of the room on myself. And now I need to start to let myself feel why. That thought makes me feel teary and alone. Dead space not empty space."

To actually hear my own words and to know that other people heard them and understood them was completely surprising. This was the first time in my life I completely identified with people whose thoughts and experiences of life were so completely like and not like my own.

I have common ground with many people and groups of people; but that commonality only goes so far. Even the people closest to me had no idea of how I really lived my life in my own mind, body and emotions. I had been looking for connection my whole life and I found a way to have it.

"I am always hiding so I can stay me. I do not know where I am hiding or what parts are hiding. I've always known I was hiding; but, I feel like I've been dropped in the middle of Dartmoor without a map and I don't know where to go. Anyone could see me; but, I can't see myself. I am starting to feel like I can move and walk, even though I don't know where I am going or what I'll say next. It's scary to feel like I'm walking on a frozen river and it might collapse at any time. I tell myself I just need to practice and put it behind me. Practice and keep going. The sun is shining."

I have spent much of my life inside of myself. I secretly hope that I haven't spent most of my life there. Quiet, away from everyone, no room for outside distraction or input. This is my hiding place. I often just sit, maybe with a quilt, often with a cat, and it looks like I'm just wasting my time. But on the inside of my brain I am in what I now know is The Nothing Place. If you have never been there, don't worry about not knowing where it is or what it is. If you have been there, please know that you will never be there alone again. We are all there with you even if you don't see us, hear us, if you don't smell us or feel us. We are all there with you. Much of my life, this retreat from the world was terrifying. I could function and go through the motions of living in the real world, but I have never felt more alone. When Pam and Anne talked about The Nothing Place, it brought up thoughts of Fright Night movies and those strangely realistic and yet gothic horror books that were so popular when I was a teenager; familiar, almost benign, and still the source of sleepless nights and nightmares.

I live in the nothing place. I am tired of clawing my way through a normal life and hanging all those disappointments on my wall. Spending hours, days, decades talking and living with people, to then be shattered when they say or do that thing that reveals they really, still, after all this time, have no clue.

I think my thoughts and make my decisions and go my own way. And I have spent lifetimes sitting in a chair feeling nothing, thinking nothing; because, nothing is better than the assumptions, accusations, and bullying that seem to arrive when I try to live in that outside world.

I know I have to live there, in the real world; but, I also know there is no place there for me. I am in the nothing place and finding that the nothing place is not empty. I am not accustomed to seeing things for me. My eyes haven't learned the frequency to see all I have in myself and so I am still learning to live in the nothing place."

By naming this place that is so familiar to me, describing the experience of being in The Nothing Place, I am able to recognize when I am there and that I can leave. "You can only heal in community." Pam said this over and over and this is my key Flourish experience. I would never have been able to confront The Nothing Place, the utter devastation and emptiness that I was living, if I hadn't trusted my classmates to be able to hold my feelings and distress when I couldn't. I trusted them to understand and I listened as they shared their own distress, heartache, and hopes for something better.

Joining this class was such a gift. We started as strangers, shy, scared, nauseous, and we became trusted compatriots. We have become friends. We all feel a belonging in this community that we built through examining our pain and our joy; our hopes and our fears; through examining what it means to be relinquished, to be given away, to be bought, to grow in silence, shame, fear, and sometimes love. To create a community through our lived experiences, to validate our core selves, and to hold a place for each other in our lives, our hopes, our joys.

I was a band geek in high school, dedicated to being the best band member I could be in the way only an obsessed teenage girl can. I was a student organizer in college. I went to lectures and protests, I taught peer classes, I studied all the literature, I talked about and volunteered with others who felt as compelled as I did to create more agency and options for people who didn't have the chance. I know what it is to throw in my lot with all of my heart and try to make a better world. I just never realized there could be a better world for me. If you had told me that spending two hours a week with other adoptees would change my life in so many ways, large and small, I would not have believed you. I wouldn't have believed I could show up that often, much less be open to examining the truth of my existence. Nothing could have convinced me that I would be a bigger person, better friend, more attentive partner, and yet, I am.

One of our last assignments was to write, draw, or sing something as a gift to another Flourisher. This prompt had a time limit. This prompt surprised me. This prompt was not like any other. This was an opportunity to acknowledge a specific person and gift them something straight from the heart. We spent some time writing, drawing, deciding what to sing and then shared our gift with each of the classmates we were assigned, one by one, as we were called on. It was fun and vulnerable writing something as a gift and sharing it with the other person. Afterwards, we were asked to write about what it was like to receive the gifts we were given.

"I was given validation, visibility, righteousness, compassion, solidarity, beauty, strength, and a certain hipness, a sophisticated coolness from my gift givers.

When I joined Flourish in August 2020, I decided I needed to do something new. For a few months I just showed up, made myself write and made myself sick when I had to read my own words out loud.

I have slowly over the last year begun to trust the process, and have begun to know Anne and Pam, to just let myself write what's in my heart and what has happened to me without the cringing fear and desperation to hide it. And I treasure every box on the screen with each of your precious faces every week and it fuels my anger that so many of us have to go through this and it fuels my love for you all and my support of you in all your you-ness.

My individual gifts are right now like precious treasures I've hidden away. But

I know one day I will make them into armor. My armor actually fits me. It was made for me and given to me with open hearts and time invested. I can choose to wear it or not.

Moving so often as a child, I would have to find new armor everywhere we went. My main choice was the shield of invisibility. After that was the cape of denial and the sword of defiance. Everywhere we moved, a new soft spot would be found and I would have to engage in the farce of forging new armor again and again.

My parents had no clue what I was talking about or experiencing and their advice was at best useless and at worst harmful. My college friends were all into be open, be free. Be yourself. Well, you may have an idea of how that would go.

But now, at 54, to be able to be me, be free, and when people shush me, challenge me, threaten me, I do live in Texas, I can stand straight in myself without questioning whether I have a right to exist. No one has earned the right to knock me down. Armor is essential, but its composition makes all the difference."

This year of living dangerously has shaken me to my core. It has made me see my own strengths, my own talents, my own dreams. I have a community that I belong to, belong in, that I trust and in which I decide every day to continue to belong. I have tools to use to help me when things are confusing and hard. I have a clearer perspective on the truth and where it exists and where it doesn't. Mostly, after a year of admitting my deepest fears and inadequacies, writing my secret hopes and dreams, of hearing the same from people like me, I see that I am normal, in that no one is normal. I feel my feet on the ground, the sun on my face, and I have every opportunity to be happy in this life.

To flourish is "to be in a vigorous state, to thrive," according to the on-line dictionary. It's been a hell of a growing season, that's for sure.

Abracadabra — It Will Be Created from my Words

Pam talked to us about wanting, that we often minimize our own wants in favor of getting by, people-pleasing, of not valuing our right to do more than just exist in the world. We were invited to want with abandon and write it all down, without thinking or examining whether it were possible. Anne gave us the prompt "Once upon a time I took a writing class and right now..."

"Once upon a time I took a writing class and right now I want a big cup of frothy, sweet coffee and a rolled croissant cinnamon roll. Then I am going to book tickets

to London, explore the Cotswolds, the Peak District, Cornwall, and take the train to Holyoke and get on the ferry to Ireland.

Then we'll fly to Hungary and explore and eat everything and then go to Austria and Germany. Along the way I will buy everything from local makers for my shop, which will be a walk in and online shop. I will start with four employees and we'll sell handmade items and coffee and baked goods.

I will also take time to write about what I see and think and feel and publish an Adoptee Travel Guide to finding your roots. This will be wildly popular so I set up a travel agency for adoptees and line up genealogists and cultural guides and language teachers and chefs and makers and adoptee certified therapists everywhere we go. There will be a studio with space for writing, photo'ing, painting, etc... to document the journey. These are not journeys for the faint of heart.

My husband and I buy a house somewhere in Europe, a little one, inexpensive, so if we lose it we're okay, and we spend more and more time outside Texas.

We travel more and eat more and write more and photograph more and visit more. We start a publishing company online to publish all the memoirs and coffee table books, the travel guides and introspections, the family trees and histories, of all the adoptees who want to share something. We have a little studio for podcasts and music and web shows.

We are so busy and happy and excited about tomorrow until, at a very auspicious age, like 111, we go to sleep and don't wake up."

I am surprised how much I crammed into a ten minute writing prompt. The practicalities of doing all the things I listed in the way I listed them is overwhelming, and the probability of all of these things happening in the way I've written them is, realistically, low. None of them are impossible and all of them may happen in some form for me, if not for a whole group of adoptees. But I can dream. I have definitely enjoyed a big cup of frothy, sweet coffee and a rolled croissant cinnamon roll. That's a good start. I have been to Dublin for a long week and enjoyed wandering the city, trying all the fish and chips and enjoying all the local brews and spirits.

I have toured the Cotswolds and the Peak District in my living room, from my old, comfy armchair, watching the television. My favorite programs are British mysteries. There is usually a memorable detective, dressed in period dress: Victorian, Edwardian, Art Deco, the war years, the post war years, the present. All time periods seem to require a civilian detective with a special talent for spotting deception. One of the best things about these shows is that they use local sites for the backdrop of the story. I've seen small English villages, the white cliffs of Dover, the inner city before and after the industrial revolution; I really think I've seen most of England, Scotland, and large pieces of Wales and Ireland without leaving home. I know it's not the same and I still enjoy it.

As to my publishing and small business successes, one step at a time. My first step was to look for the helpers. I found Anne Heffron and Pam Cordano and thanks to these two women I found my community. Community is where you can be safe enough and brave enough and big enough to dream. That was a big step, and what will the next step be? I don't know, but I know it will be in my community, with my people. I want to sew a flag and write a community constitution. Our anthem is going to be great! Anyone else out there interested?

Maybe, once this pandemic is over, we will travel again and I can make some of this dream come true. Right now, I'm sitting at my computer, writing this essay and enjoying the fact that my words are being read by you, right now. You are now part of making my dream come true. I hope I have encouraged you to dream as big as you want, as specific or as broad as you dare. It's time we played the central role in our own dreams, our own lives. Wouldn't it be magic?

I Am

I am a person who is creative

with an unpredictable way of thinking and

hard to get to know.

Normal, almost invisible in ubiquity on the outside.

I am a Tardis.

The strong is on the inside.

On the inside

worlds,

lives,

ideas,

thoughts

that can only grow so big because on the outside

trust is so small.

This is not a story about Truth as you know it.

No one gave honesty and I don't owe anyone honesty.

I am not a judge or juror and neither are you.

I am not in the business of convincing or persuading you.

I am not

and should never have been

a business.

I am a person who is creative

with an unpredictable way of thinking and

hard to get to know.

DAWN'S STORY:

I was born Baby Girl Bryant. Bryant was a fictitious name to disguise a uniquely Hungarian last name. Relinquished at birth, I lived in a foster home for two months until I was adopted through a state agency. I grew up an only child and I have always known I was adopted. I lived in a military family and I attended 10 different schools before graduating high school. My biological father died in 1995 and never knew about me, as far as I can tell. I am not in reunion with anyone in my biological family.

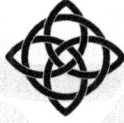

DOMINICA SELVAGGIO, LMHC, NCC

OREGON AND HAWAII

(THEY/THEM)

Freedom to Flourish

IT IS OCTOBER OF 2020. I sit in a mid-century modern orange rocking chair in the corner of my bedroom in my vintage Portland apartment. This chair is a great source of comfort and a place that I find myself passing many hours staring and daydreaming and smoking spliffs (a mixture of cannabis and tobacco) out of the singular, old, white wooden paned window that has a view of the sprawling courtyard below.

I am not well. No, I am unwell. I am in a state of dis-ease. I can hardly feel that I have a body with legs tucked underneath me. I can hardly feel the edge of my ribs as they jut out of my center with every shallow breath. I am hardly here. I am hardly awake. I am hardly living.

The sounds of flash bangs and helicopters paint the soundscape in the distance. At this point, I barely notice the flinches and shudders my body makes in response. There is a crackling electric tension in the smoke that shakes in the air in response to all of the noise. There are many spirits passing through the ether. A death a minute below me beneath me above me surrounding me. There are the Black Lives Matter protests and kidnappings by the National Guard and wildfires and the coughs of those sick with Covid-19 coloring this landscape. I cannot tell the difference between the cannabis and tobacco embers I inhale and the ashes of the dead trees and plants and animals carried in the winds through my window.

But there is the orange chair to hold me. The orange chair that I bought from a white family in the suburbs of Seattle a year ago for my first studio apartment to call my own as a 30-year-old adult human. The orange chair that the Black baby that the white couple adopted crawled on happily, unwanting to say goodbye to its vibrant hue when it came time for me to take it and leave. The Black baby separated from its biological mother and family to be raised by people who share no genetic or skin links. I felt remorse buying this chair once I saw the way this child loved it so. The color orange is a color of psychic protection. And I prayed for that baby to be given the protection it needed from the violence of white assimilation and adoption as I drove away, chair in tow.

And now I am the one who needs protection. From the thoughts and feelings of self hate and disgust and shame and loneliness and despair and grief that propel me to seek seek seek relief anywhere but inside of myself. Anywhere but the hollow shell I have become through my constant running and avoidance of what aches. I can't eat. I can't sleep. I can't do anything but sit in this chair and daydream and listen to the voices coming from my iPad screen and let my pen move when given writing prompts I am not certain I can complete.

The voices mostly sound like far off echoes, but somehow the words of other adult adoptees speaking and sharing their writing brings me enough back into my body to be able to share my own words when prompted. I am in a group called Flourish, facilitated by Anne and Pam, the two women who hosted the first adoptee healing retreat I ever went to back in August of 2019 in New Jersey. That retreat was the first time I was able to really name and feel the full impact of the trauma of being separated from my mother and placed in foster care at the age of four, and then being adopted at the age of 10. The ways this trauma had fragmented and separated my mind from my body and fragmented my spirit. Fragmented my soul. I feel less a living human and more a mosaic without glue to cement the pieces. More a constellation of broken parts that form a moving shape shifting picture. I can be anything you need as long as you don't ask me to be me.

Over time, as I sit week to week in my orange chair, staring at my iPad screen, daring myself to write, daring myself to be seen by other adoptees, something starts to shift in me. I don't feel so alone and I don't feel so crazy in my own brain. Even as I was faced with an unfair eviction attempt based in disability discrimination (my landlords were trying to force me out so they could charge more money for the unit I was renting), even as I was rapidly losing form and losing weight because I could not bring myself to eat (my body was living in a constant hyper vigilant and contracted state), even as the protests and wildfires raged, even as my new relationship with a sweet and kind woman was dissolving because of all of the stress, even as I consumed spliff after spliff, cigarette after cigarette, even as I spiraled into the deepest pit of despair – I felt held. I felt seen.

I felt mirrored by this virtual group called Flourish. A verb I had never imagined could be true for myself.

The magic of having other adoptees mirror my pain started to slowly but surely shift something inside of me. Little by little, I began to care more and more about my well being. Yes, I was in crisis. Yes, I was held. After a friend of mine expressed concern for my weight loss over coffee one day, I knew that something had to change. The eviction attempt ended up being a blessing in disguise because it propelled me forward to look for help for what I was now able to recognize as a relapse in the eating disorder I thought I had defeated in my youth. I started to consider my options for treatment. I could stay in Portland, a city I felt very little emotional connection to. A city plagued by clouds and rain and polarization and violence. A city I only ended up in because of circumstances outside of my control (the pandemic). Or. Or. Or. I could go to a treatment center in Hawaii, called Ai'Pono, which means "to nourish with ease."

I entered residential treatment in Hawaii for Anorexia and Avoidant Restrictive Food Intake Disorder (ARFID) in November of 2020. I spent exactly 30 days being contained in an imperfect place being forced to sit at a table six times a day and stare down my biggest fear. Nourishment. Food. Living. Life. This was no easy feat, given that I myself am an eating disorder therapist and it was so painful to be back in the seat of client instead of clinician. I felt so much shame for needing the help. But even throughout treatment, I stayed connected with my Flourish family. I got special permission to attend these adoptee support groups amidst the regimented schedule that is living in an inpatient mental health facility.

Having an eating disorder is akin to slow suicide. You've probably read the stat many times in the essays in this book before mine, but it bears repeating. Adoptees are four times more likely than non-adopted people to attempt suicide. Another way to say that is that adoption has a 25 percent death rate. Adoptees are also far more likely to struggle with eating disorders, addiction, PTSD, depression, anxiety, and ADHD than non-adopted folks. People don't like to acknowledge this painful truth in our culture. It goes directly against the dominant narrative that adoption is a way to "save" kids and a good way to start a family if you are unable to have your own. Adoption didn't save me. I did. My fellow adoptees did.

I write these words now, sitting in a pink velvet chair in the office of my Oahu apartment in February of 2022. I read recently that pink is the color of playfulness, love, romance, and tenderness. I feel comforted by this color in the wake of yet another romantic relationship ending that by some miraculous energy, I did not initiate. I say this because most of the relationships I have had in my adult life have come to an end by my own avoidant hands. I used to find the feeling of true intimacy intolerable. No, not intolerable – torturous. To allow myself to be seen and known and loved used to be a special kind of hell that somehow was worse to my adoptee brain than the hell of isolation and disconnection. But that wasn't true this time – this time I was the one equipped to stay, and unfortunately, my partner was not. And don't get me wrong – I am grieving, but I don't feel shattered the way I would have had it not been for the year of sitting with other adoptees and healing in Flourish. In fact, I feel more whole and integrated and capable of holding and being present with all of my emotions in a way that I simply was unable to do before this year of community support.

Recently, I went through a guided psychedelic healing session that allowed me to access the four-year-old part of me that was still living in the dirty apartment in the suburbs of Chicago that I got taken by the police from. That child part of me has been living in this apartment in my mind since the cataclysmic separation from my mother occurred. Just curled up in the fetal position in an unkempt bunk bed in a dark room waiting for mom to come home. The child doesn't live there alone in that apartment anymore. All of the adult adoptees and Anne and Pam in Flourish helped them leave. I helped them leave. Now they have been transformed into a Blue Jay bird, free to fly and soar and nest where they please. Freedom to Flourish outside of The Nothing Place. Free to feel everything without needing to numb or escape the pain.

It feels worth mentioning that other changes have occurred as a result of participating in this group. I am fully weight restored and have maintained my recovery for more than a little over a year now. I have returned to my work as Licensed Mental Health Counselor. I am studying psychedelic assisted therapy, realizing that most of my child and adult life was spent in a semi-psychedelic dissociative state called "The Nothing Place." I feel equipped to guide others through and out of this place. I started a podcast interviewing other transgender and non-binary folks about their relationships with food and body and nourishment. I fell in love. I got rejected and abandoned by that love. It hurt, it still hurts, but I didn't fall apart. I have a sense of community and belonging on the island that I now call home. I am sober. Fully in reality. Fully in my body. Fully allowed to be exactly as I am.

And in case you were wondering, my beloved orange chair still lives in the storage unit in Portland where I put all of my belongings when I decided to take the mega leap to seek help in Hawaii last year. Someday soon, I will go back and clear out the cobwebs and the ghosts of that difficult time. I will sell what I no longer need, what I cannot easily ship to my new home on this island of ease. I will release what no longer serves me. I will keep what nourishes me. I will root root root into my new found sense of Ai'Pono. Ease in nourishment. I wish this feeling for all adoptees.

A final thank you to all of my fellow group members in Flourish and to Anne and Pam for creating such a special container for us to heal together in. I may not always be the most participatory, but please know how deeply you have impacted my life and how much I love you.

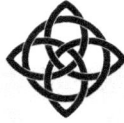

EVAN BROOK

CALIFORNIA

Riffing on "Grandma's Hands" by Bill Withers

BILL WITHERS' SOFT, SIMPLE, nearly spiritual song "Grandma's Hands" always brings me solace and feelings of acceptance and community. From the opening rhythmic *chitsh* of the high hat, I immediately feel my thundering heart begin to slow and sync first with the high hat, then slowing further to align with the heartbeat sounds of the snare drum. I have loved this song for the soothing effect it has on me since first I heard it. Once I listened to the lyrics – about the gifts offered by a beloved Grandma through her sometimes aching and swollen, but always loving hands – I was gone.

Sometimes I feel as though I have sought all my life for hands – hands that could comfort, nurture, lift up and protect. When I entered this world, I waited to be received by hands I would innately recognize, but they did not appear. They did not cradle me, hold me against their warm skin, or check that all my appendages were counted and recounted with silent wonder. Instead, I was handed into the arms of strangers who didn't smell or sound familiar. It was into those hands I was expected to settle. I can almost see tiny hands grasping at the air in confusion, searching for that bonded connection and coming up empty. I have a distinct memory of meeting my adoptive grandfather and grandmother when I was two years old. The plump arms of my granny enfolded me, cooing with pleasure. Her hugs felt like being enveloped in a warm and substantial cloud. This is the closest I can imagine to the Grandma of the song. In contrast, my lone impression of my grandfather was of his hard, bony, cold and unwelcoming hand when I reached for it. I can't locate any memories of being hugged by my adoptive parents as I was by my grandmother. Perhaps the distance of a generation made holding an unwanted child easier. Or perhaps my grandmother simply had never met an unwanted child.

Ridiculous as it may sound, I have no idea whether she knew that I was adopted, so deeply unspoken was the topic in my home.

In Bill Withers' song, the Grandma offers cautionary advice to a playful child and steps in to prevent a beating. Never does she scold or punish the child for simply being a child. In my adoptive home, I was expected to act like a small adult. Raised as an only child, I found few opportunities to play. To my memory, my granny visited us in California only one other time which coincided with Halloween. With my granny, I could act like a child with impunity. I even have pictures of me sitting on her lap in my Halloween costume. She has one arm wrapped around me and a hand steadying me. I was dressed as the devil and had a candy cigarette dripping from my lip. I couldn't say whether I or my adoptive parents selected the costume. I know I bedeviled the hell out of them and was a constant source of aggravation.

If only we could pass down gifts of nurturance, compassion and protection rather than the trauma that is adoption. In the end, it is that very human need for love, connection and belonging that is at the center of both the wounding and the healing.

Discovery Melancholy

When I first became aware that I was adopted, I was about seven years old. I was full of questions, as one is at that age. While my adoptive parents were patient in answering my endless streams of questions on many topics, on the subject of my adoption they were consistently and uniformly tight-lipped. When I inquired about the circumstances of my adoption, or asked for information about my birth parents, I was stonewalled. Occasionally, my curiosity was met with platitudes such as "They were just like us." What did that mean? Caucasian? Presbyterian? A doctor and a nurse/housewife? Southerners? It meant nothing to me. The more ways I tried to get around the great wall they had erected between me and this information, the more lidded glances were exchanged; the more pinched became their expressions. Eventually, inevitably, my mother would burst into tears, sobbing "We're your parents!" and the discussion, such as it was, was concluded.

To my mind, if the fortress my parents erected around my adoption information and their staunch defense of its perimeter were so necessary, something truly terrible and unpleasant must reside inside. The belief that I landed on was that I simply wasn't wanted. The newborn me had done something horrendous, so reprehensible, by virtue of my birth that my biological parents could not and would not keep me. As painful as this thought was, it conveniently kept me well-within the narrative that suited my adoptive parents – that I was "lucky" that they adopted me. It kept me in lock-step as the good child, the small adult, lest I repeat my sins and be shipped off again.

Although it wasn't constantly present in my mind, I lived with the certain knowledge that, if I had done something so terrible once, I might unwittingly do so again, especially since I had no idea what that thing might have been.

I carried these beliefs with me throughout my childhood. I stopped asking questions. I didn't look for the truth about my adoption until after both my adoptive parents had died. Finally, there was no one left who could give me away for bad behavior. I submitted a DNA kit and impatiently waited weeks for the results to post. I browsed my heritage – still white, northern European with some Scandinavian influence. My North American relatives were concentrated in the South. Nothing really newsworthy there. Then, squirming a bit, I opened the genetic matches section and found instant relatives, a whole family-full, though over time they proved as unforthcoming as my adoptive parents. I poured over my siblings' family tree, having to consciously remind myself that it was, in some way, my family tree too. Trying to piece together a narrative without their help, I cycled through story after story, modifying each version to fit some new piece of data I had gleaned through genealogy, public records or combing newspaper archives. I kept hoping to find a back door into the family, a corner puzzle piece on which I could begin to hang the branches of my own family history.

Through my online searching, I found the eulogy of my biological father, and with it a smorgasbord of family photos, fifty or more, showing all manner of people who were strangers to me. Wrestling with the queasy feeling of being an internet stalker, I liberally decorated my sibling's family tree with photos, trying to link names on the tree to the faces in the photos. I tried on stories in which my mother was sent to California to get rid of an unwanted pregnancy so that she could return to Alabama to marry well in her family's eyes. Or that my birth father simply hadn't known about me, and that my mother had no choice but to relinquish me. I found that version mildly comforting as it didn't require them to have rejected me per se. It was the Baby Scoop Era, after all. It's what was done.

After weeks of searching genealogical trees and newspaper stories, I uncovered a piece of information that simultaneously stopped me cold, took my breath and replaced it with a hot, twisting, sickening discomfort. My birth parents had become engaged mere weeks after I was born and married several months later.

With this discovery, I came crashing back to the story I created as a child – my birth parents hadn't wanted me. I was a problem to be handled. Wrong.

Unworthy. Unlovable. How could they give up a child – me – and announce their engagement to each other only two weeks later? How could they then go on to have two more children – my full biological siblings – and say nothing? This version of the story continued to haunt me until I obtained my Non-Identifying Information from the state of California.

In states like California, where my closed adoption occurred, I could request Non-Identifying Information*, whereas access to my original birth certificate remains prohibited. When I requested and received these censored and fragmented documents, in which names and identifying information related to my birth parents were redacted, it felt furtive and demeaning. Adoption secrecy feels overbearing, paternalistic and offensive.

My Non-Identifying Information paints a somewhat different picture of my relinquishment and subsequent adoption with which I am still finding my way. Based on these documents, my adoptive parents actually met with my birth mother, at the least, and perhaps both my birth parents. This news served to electrify the fortress they had constructed and defended throughout my childhood as if my birth parents were actually inside the fortress which, in a sense, they were.

My parents had MET them. Another bombshell in these documents was that my birth mother seemed reticent to give me up and that she reached out to the individual who arranged my adoption to check on me months afterward. This news still feels jagged, like it could rip me open. The birth mother I believed all my life didn't want me, was actually concerned about me.

Not enough to keep me, look for me, or even tell her other biological children about me, but at least enough to call and check on me. It might seem like a bread crumb but, to me it feels like a feast.

It is gut-wrenching that I have only now received this information, nearly six decades after I was relinquished. It is appalling that I have to tiptoe through genealogical trees, skulk through newspaper graveyards, and beg the state for information that is rightfully mine to learn my own damn history. Had I learned this information earlier, I might have searched sooner or pushed harder with my sibling to meet my birth mother while she was still alive. Although it would no doubt have upset my siblings' perception of their family and their (our) parents, it might have brought me and my mother some modicum of healing. That adoptive parents can believe that keeping information from their children is somehow safer, kinder and healthier for all concerned mystifies me. That governments assume such archaic, patriarchal positions which keep adult individuals from their own vital information is criminal. Closed adoption and the myriad ways in which an adoptee's origin and identity are kept from them is simply cruel.

*In states in which closed adoptions occur, Non-Identifying Information is what the state discloses to adoptees in lieu of providing access to our original birth certificate or the details of our adoption. It may contain information about biological parents and the adoption process used. Names and identifying information are redacted. Requesting and receiving these censored and fragmented documents feels furtive and demeaning; the adoption secrecy they represent feels overbearing, paternalistic and offensive.

On Finding Language, Voice and Community

My appetite for the stories and voices of fellow adoptees is virtually insatiable. Week after week, our shared writings have offered new language for feelings and experiences that, for me, long have been wordless. Our stories are powerful, moving, startling, unsettling, inspiring, funny and comforting. Our voices are unique, creative, lyrical, raw and undeniably vibrant. Listening to the shared writings each week has been a gift for the senses and an embrace for all of the lost children in me.

For me as a writer, each week brought challenges – to dig into my experiences and feelings, to face putting often difficult words to the writing prompts that reflect me or something I have to say. Often so much of my life as an adoptee has been lived in shame and silent secrecy. An adoptee writing group feels antithetical to this legacy like a well-aimed searchlight. Each week writing for me has functioned like a poorly constructed pipe bomb, razing the roof on the house that adoption built and flooding it with light. It feels like a revolutionary act.

What has been invaluable to me has been the experience of showing up, reaching and writing, sharing, and then listening. Listening to the other adoptee writers has been such a pleasure and felt so very validating. When adoptees give voice to our experiences, it exposes and dismantles the crippling façade of the cheerful adoption narrative. That is something I can get behind and to which I would lend my developing voice.

Evan's Story:

> I was adopted at birth through private arrangement and raised as an only child. I have known that I was adopted since I was about seven years old. Through DNA testing, I located biological family. Unfortunately, both of my biological parents died before we could meet. My remaining family members – siblings, an uncle, nieces and nephews – are not open to contact. What name my birth parents might have given me is unknown as my adoption record and birth certificate remain sealed by the state of California.
>
> Evan is my chosen name.

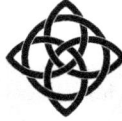

FRANCINE J BAUER (APRIL GAULKE)
FLORIDA

I FOUND OUT I WAS ADOPTED when I was around nine years old. My friend told me. In my nine-year-old head, if nobody was talking about adoption in my own house, it must be a dirty secret. This has shaped and warped me to who I am today. Woven into every fiber of my being. The damage is irreparable and true.

I started searching for birth family in the early 1990's when I was in my 30's and newly diagnosed with cancer. Over the past 30 years, I have eventually found everyone: Birth mother, birth father, half-sister Dee, who has passed. Half-brother John, who has also passed but I sadly never got to meet. My heart, my half-sister Joyce. A surprise half-sister, Drue, from my birth father's side. And three years ago, I was finally reunited with my full sister, Sari. It does my heart no good to dwell on the years we've lost together, how different our lives would have been. We all know the pain. The damage is irreparable and true.

My Flourish family has given me strength, courage, beauty and insight. We have cried together and laughed at adoptee shit that no one else can understand. We've grieved together and grown to have a deep respect and love for each other. I've started using my birth name, April, trying it on to see if it still fits. I'm in awe of this group of beautiful souls and their generosity of spirit to always be available to any of us in need. Our collective experiences have changed my life this past year. I've built long-lasting relationships and these friends and experiences have become part of my truth.

FRANCINE'S STORY:

I was born in Hollywood, Florida. My birth parents Phyllis, who was 28 years old, and Bill, who was 30 years old, were married, had stable jobs, a house and a sailboat. He was the love of her life. Bill was a jazz musician who was reassembling the pipe organ from the Coconut Grove Playhouse. No room for a baby. I was the youngest of Phyllis' five children, none of which she was raising. Phyllis and Bill met in high school where Phyllis proceeded to get pregnant. Her first baby girl, born in 1949, was put up for adoption. Phyllis had three more children before abandoning them for Bill. After my birth, I was named April and then left in the hospital for two weeks while the financials were agreed upon and a private adoption was finalized. My name was changed to Francine, after my adoptive father. The damage is irreparable and true.

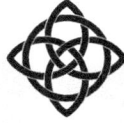

GLORYA JEAN

CALIFORNIA

My Year in Flourish

SOMETIME IN NOVEMBER OF 2020 I heard there was going to be a group of adoptees meeting weekly for the next year. The group would be discussing and writing about their experiences with adoption. Something told me to do it, although I couldn't begin to imagine doing anything with a group of strangers on a weekly basis, let alone for an entire year. Discussing adoption sounded both emotionally terrifying and hopefully healing.

My birth father, who I had been in reunion with for two years, had recently died and the world was dealing with the pandemic. My children and grandchildren were living an hour away. People in my immediate family were extremely high risk so I'd seen no more than the same seven people for almost an entire year. Like so much of the world I was depressed and incredibly lonely.

I saw a comment on an Instagram post about Flourish and reached out to the anonymous adoptee who made the comment. They replied quickly full of excitement and nothing but good things to say about the open meetings they had attended. Their reply was enough for me to sign up. I told myself I would stick the year out no matter what.

I needed this group.

The first Wednesday night that we met I was filled with nervous excitement. I looked around the Zoom screen at a group of strangers. It's doubtful that any of us were comfortable. Over the next few weeks I tried to reach out to a few people and got some short replies in return. I took it as a sign that they didn't really like me and thought that maybe I should quit the group. I felt like I didn't belong. In reality, we were all still feeling the whole thing out. It was sad to me that several weeks in, it still seemed to me that, even though we were all vulnerable, open, and honest, we continued to feel like strangers. Every single week I had to force myself to sign on. While I felt like the outcast of my youth there was something that lured me back each week.

Quite often the writing prompts were difficult for me to write. I found myself trying to scribble out coherent sentences while trying to break a lifetime of silence on feelings and thoughts I had rarely, if ever, allowed myself to speak. Writing the prompts also caused me to think, all week long in fact. As each adoptee read their writing aloud I would hear the others verbalize things that I had experienced or thought my entire life. Oftentimes, someone would put words to a lifelong feeling that I, myself, had never had words for. Almost every week I would have tears streaming down my face, usually in relief, often in shame. My heart broke for each of us. The honesty was staggering. I truly can't remember a time in my life where I have been around people who were so open and honest with their thoughts, let alone hearing what adoptees felt about their lives. So often we would see everyone shaking their heads in agreement as one of us would read aloud the secret thoughts we had held in our entire lives. At times I was overwhelmed at learning we all felt the same way or had the exact same experience in a totally different life. I can't tell you how healing it was to know that while we all lived feeling so alone in our experience, we never were. Other adoptees were right there with us. Feeling the same way. If only we had known.

I set up a Facebook group for us to post on during the week. We found it a great way to get to know each other even better. After the group ended on Wednesday nights, whoever could make it would meet over Facetime for an hour or two. The discussions and connections we made during those hours were essential to my healing. I believe that the others who made it would agree.

Week after week we met and bared our souls but I began to wonder if we would ever really come together in the way that I was hoping. As usual, the adoptee in me believed that they just didn't like me. In my head I imagined everyone texting each other during the week and developing these great relationships. Everyone but me. Maybe they were. Maybe they weren't.

After this year with adoptees, I can honestly say that it's not just me. We often feel alone, out of place and unwanted. Many of us, myself included, felt we were a burden. There are times I still feel like the group doesn't like me. I know that isn't true, but I still wrestle with that feeling that was planted in my brain the day my mother gave me away. Fortunately, I know now that it's a feeling we all share.

One night in March one of us, themselves a therapist, mentioned that we needed a short closing so we could leave the emotion of the meetings behind. Most nights ended abruptly and emotionally charged. Members of the group all seemed to really need and want this, yet the leaders did not. I can barely remember the discussion as it was horribly uncomfortable not just for me, but for others. Some people couldn't even look at their screen; a few may even have turned off their camera. Voices were raised. People spoke over each other and emotions were high. The discussion came to a complete halt when they were shut down. We realized we really did not have any say in our group. It wasn't even our group. It was the leaders group and that was that. The members of the group chatted off line later that night and the days following. That was when we truly came together as a family. I likened the experience to what I suppose a family with close siblings goes through. There are times parents discipline the kids and send them to their room. When the kids get together they'd talk about how the parents weren't listening to them and were treating them unfairly. It felt like that. We came together and stayed together after that. We became solid to the core.

Even though I loved the group I still had to convince myself to sign on each week. It was a bit like going to the gym. You know you're going to have a good time and feel better in the end, but getting in your car and driving there is tough. Or is that just me? I truly cared about every single person in the group and I was feeling closer to many members of the group. I finally felt like I was beginning to make some friends, it just wasn't happening as quickly as I was hoping for.

Each week we continued getting to know each other as we would take turns exposing our deepest, darkest truths during the group. We found out that nearly every single one of us had felt as if we didn't belong in our adoptive families, we felt like no one truly loved us as children, we thought of suicide throughout our lives, we were all lonely even when we were surrounded by others, and so much more.

Summer, along with catastrophe, came to my life. Tony, my 33-year-old stepson, was found dead of an overdose. He had wrestled with schizoaffective (schizophrenia and bi-polar) disorder and drug addiction for more than 10 years. While we always knew the day would come, we never expected it to show up that day. We were devastated. Tony had been my son since he was six. How do you survive the loss of a child? I felt comforted by the fact that I had this wonderful group of people that understood me.

Grief is so weird. We adoptees have spent our entire lives grieving. Even when we didn't know that we were grieving, we were. Surely, this group would know what I needed. They of all people would realize that this was yet another abandonment; that's the adoptee brain for you. I hoped that as adoptees they would see me. I was mostly let down and it hurt more than I could have imagined. Adoption. The gift that keeps on giving.

I had to remind myself that as an adoptee I either expect too little or too much from others. Having worked in the business of grief, I knew what to expect when you lose a child. Death is hard enough. People don't know what to say or do. They scatter. I needed more than people could give and I let it affect me. Like most adoptees I either wouldn't or couldn't ask for help, nor could I show that I even needed or wanted it. I was fine. I'm always fine. Sadly, I let my feelings of disappointment and sadness get to me.

Fall came and my father in law, a man I really loved for nearly 30 years, lost his life to Covid-19. I expected to at least get a text, email, anything really, from one or both of the leaders at some point, saying they were sorry I had lost not just one family member, but two.

Nothing.

At one point a member's dog had to be put to sleep. An absolutely devastating decision. My heart ached for her and her family. The leaders asked for a moment of silence. I was crushed. While I ached for her awful loss all I could think was, "Where was Tony's moment of silence?" There were other members who had also lost loved ones. Where was their moment of silence? I was furious. I'll be forever thankful when that sweet member, who in her grief, spoke up and said she didn't think it was appropriate. I would never have thought any less of her if we had done it, but in that moment I saw how much she cared about the rest of us.

My grief was extremely heavy.

I felt slighted by the leadership. I was missing more meetings. When I did show up, I wasn't really present. I felt my grief was ignored. Looking back, I ignored it most of all. The adoptee in me hoped that I would be missed but I felt like I wasn't. I had thought the leaders would reach out to see if I was okay. They, themselves, were adoptees. As the saying goes, "Expectations are premeditated resentments." Another lesson learned. Our adoptee brains can really pull some tricks on us. People had their own lives, their own troubles. Some have since said they felt they would be bothering me. I let it get to me. I was broken. At times I was in an absolute rage over it. I decided to leave the group. I know better than to stay where I'm not wanted.

My close friends in the group reminded me it was bigger than the leaders, that it was about the group. It's true, the members were why I was truly there. Really. I loved and cared for every one of these people, even the leaders. If I left, what was that going to do? To them? To me? I'm an expert at cutting off my nose to spite my face.

So where I had once been proud that I had not missed our weekly meetings, I started to skip more and more of them. The last half of the year I questioned if I'd be able to attend each month while I was also getting an email reminder that I still needed to pay. That would have been the perfect time for them to ask if I was okay or letting me know that I was missed. I continued to pay for meetings I wasn't even attending. Each week I would sit in front of my screen, in tears, willing myself to sign on but couldn't bring myself to press enter. Other times I signed on and within minutes, I would sign off. It was too difficult to sit there while I was filled with rage and sorrow. Losing this group was another loss. Not wanting to be a burden to anyone, I kept my unbearable sadness to myself.

Unfortunately or perhaps fortunately, there were others with their own trials and concerns. What group is ever without them? I am one of the adoptees in the group that just so happens to have another member of the group who lives in the same town. While I had thought of reaching out to them to set up a lunch or something I thought I'd be a bother. As luck would have it, they invited me! I quickly accepted and we became fast friends. If there is one thing I am beyond thankful for, it's them. Their friendship was a life-ring in the stormy sea.

As painful and as full of loss as this year was, being in a true community with adoptees added so much to my life. As adoptees, we grow up without any mirroring which is so very important. Listening to other adoptees honestly share their innermost thoughts helped, not just me, but all of us, to experience true Emotional Mirroring for the very first time. I'm so grateful for this experience and for the vulnerability of people who started out as total strangers but who are now friends for life. I would do anything for any of them, they're like family.

These are the friends I had been praying for. I text or video chat with many of them throughout the week. Some of us talk on the phone at all hours of the night and day. Not a day goes by that we don't hear from someone in the group. We can have the most honest conversations. There is never a reason to worry that we won't know what we're talking about; there is no need to explain. We just get it. I am thrilled to have met several members over the last few months. Recently I went out of town for the weekend with three other members to celebrate our Milestone birthdays together! It was a magical birthday that I never could have imagined had I not spent the year with these people.

While I started out the year feeling lost and lonely, I finished feeling happier than I've been in years. If it wasn't for the emotional mirroring, I don't think I would have started taking better care of my emotional and mental health. I started seeing a therapist to deal with adoption trauma and CPTSD. I was introduced to the life changing 5 Rhythms Dance which has become a near daily practice. I've become certified in Neurographic Drawing and I even joined a bowling team! I'm working out at a gym several times a week and I'm even thinking of starting yoga up again; it's been years. For the first time in many years I can say I am really, truly happy. It's a great place to be!

This year we are meeting without leaders. They have moved on to help other adoptees. We still meet every week and now it's like we've known each other forever. It's getting much easier to not feel like we're bothering each other, to ask for help when we need it and to be honest with what we're thinking, not just in our group, but out in the world as well. We know we don't ever have to explain or apologize. We will always see everyone nod their heads in agreement and understanding, and we'll hear back, "yes, I've felt that way too. "

I was able to end the year, as I set out, still a member of this group. The year was messy, difficult and full of drama, but isn't every year? I found true introspection, lots of laughter, and remarkable friendships. My year in Flourish was an amazing year of growth. More than I could imagine. I've learned so much about myself and adoptees, in general. We're all on a healing journey. While most of us felt alone and unseen, even in the adoptee reflection, we've learned we're not alone. At all.

A Letter from North American Adoption Agencies, LLC

Dear Flourish Adoptee Group,

We can't believe you have the audacity to write to us. It's bad enough you've been trying to expose our billion dollar industry. We truly regret that you have begun calling us out publicly. As the self appointed representative for those who are making money selling children by adoption we must insist that you put a halt to your actions.

Of course, we've never taken single women seriously. No one ever took women seriously until recently and really, you all have a long way to go. We may say we care about mothers and families, but adoptees and birthmothers know this isn't true. As for caring about babies and children, you are right, we should care about them. Let's just say most people think we do and that's good enough for us. We never actually considered that what we were doing was the wrong thing. Really, we didn't care. We still don't. We wish we could say it wasn't all about the money - but it's all about the money. It always has been.

After a bit of discussion we can see that you adoptees have a point. Adoption is, as you say, really screwed up. What made us think that taking an infant from their mother was okay? While we don't allow kittens, puppies, goats or horses to be taken from their mothers it didn't seem like human babies would actually suffer. Why would they? We believed that you all would just blend in. Why wouldn't you? We spoke with some adoptive mothers, they say it's not their fault. Just try harder.

You say that we have ruined the lives of millions of children and some of their mothers. You say you're depressed, obsessed, and suicidal. That's too bad. We really plan on continuing with the same old thing. Sure we will make a few changes so that the public will believe we are doing the right thing and you'll all continue to look like you are ungrateful or just had a bad experience. There are too many people that insist they need to have children, and quite frankly, there is way too much money at stake.

We have discussed your list of suggestions or -demands. For you to request that adoptees -have access to their original birth certificates, genetic makeup, medical history and a lifetime of paid healthcare and therapy, that would cost us more money than we would ever be willing to spend. You should be able to pull yourselves together and focus more on being grateful.

Please discontinue your inflammatory posts on social media. You are making adoptive parents upset. Apparently, the adoptive parents are afraid that younger adoptees will start asking uncomfortable questions. You know that is the least of their worries. Your posts are also upsetting couples undergoing fertility treatments. Some of them are beginning to question if adoption should actually be their last resort. We need these people. We have vacation homes and extended vacations in Europe planned.

Get on with your lives.

Sincerely,

Uve Wasted Urtime

President

North American Adoption Agencies LLC.

From My Notebook

2/2021

How can you be your authentic self when people thought they were buying a Barbie doll and ended up with a generic doll? My adoptive mother wanted, no... she *expected* perfection. She adopted a blue-eyed, blond-haired baby girl. As my hair darkened she would buy all kinds of blonding shampoos to try to extend the life of her blond-haired child. The message to six-year-old me was I wasn't okay the way I was. Puberty brought out a head full of curls that she really couldn't stand. She insisted I keep my hair short. Every haircut would result in my parents teasing me and calling me George. They'd say I looked ugly and my father would insist I looked like a boy. They were disappointed they didn't get a Barbie and I've been disappointed I'll never be one.

2/2021

I was one person with my adopted family and another person when away from my family. I thought I was comfortable with who I was. Now that I am mostly out of the fog and in reunion I don't know who the hell I am any more. I'm not sure I even have the energy to figure it out.

3/2021

Upper limit (issues)

The book, *The Big Leap*, by Gay Hendricks writes about upper limit problems and how we sabotage ourselves to keep ourselves comfortable.

As an adoptee, I feel I have -fundamental flaws and early on I decided that they're true.

1. Fatal flaw – I'm unlovable
2. Disloyal – being disloyal to parents, siblings, relatives, etc.
3. I'm a burden – if I become more... I'm a burden to the world.
4. Outshine – Don't outshine people because it will make them feel bad and they won't like you.

*I wasn't loveable, let alone likeable.

*Even though -my parents tried to keep me tied to and dependent on them, I've always felt like a burden. Saying that makes me feel that I'm still disloyal to my parents and they're dead.

*Being in reunion makes me feel disloyal to dead people.

*I've been thinking of quitting Flourish because of upper limit problems. But today made me think - where else will I find a group of such incredibly courageous people? Where else can I be soooo honest and free?

What's not okay for me right now?

It's not okay that I always feel like an outsider and that no one likes me. I feel like I often say the wrong thing. I still often feel like I'm a burden.

It's not okay that my parents drilled into my head how ugly I am. It's not okay that I have a hard time looking at myself or taking pictures. I can't stand to see myself in pictures. It's not okay that now that I'm older I feel even more insecure. I shouldn't care what others think of me. It's not okay that I don't feel comfortable in my own body and barely even in my soul. I really just want to be happy with myself.

What's not okay is that our son is dead.

What's going okay for me right now?

For the first time in my life I'm taking care of myself.

I'm beginning to do the things I really want to do.

I'm starting to put myself as a priority. I'm learning to set better boundaries.

I'm taking care of my mental and emotional health.

9/2021

Prompt: My dream for our group.

My dream is that each of us never feel alone. I dream we never doubt ourselves or our worth. I dream we can make peace with our pasts and the lives that never were. I dream each of us knows that at least one of us is always available to talk. That we have lasting friendships. That we remember our relationships with each other are solid and that we understand each other like no other group does. Most of all, I dream that our hearts are truly healed.

9/2021

Moms will kill for their children. Ours must let us go, and we were exchanged for a price. Caged and tamed for the happiness and entertainment of others.

Random Notes

Have less guilt in choosing you. – Coleen

If you're worried about losing people in your life you've already lost them. – Unknown

Control is a substitute for trust! – Unknown

We traded our honesty for safety. – Unknown

The authentic life is in no way easier. – Monique

GLORYA JEAN'S STORY:

I was born in 1962 which makes me part of the Baby Scoop Era (1945-1973) when 1.5 million girls and women were sent off to maternity homes to deliver their babies in secret. According to my Non-Identifying information and information I found during my 20-year search my Birthmother turned 18-years old two weeks after I was born. Using a fake name and other information when she was admitted to the hospital allowed her to leave the hospital a week later. She fully intended to keep and raise me. We somehow ended up 205 miles away where she was arrested on a petty charge. While in jail she was convinced to relinquish me. She came to see me twice after making that decision. I was adopted between the age of four months and six months and legally adopted soon after. I have no idea where I was or who was caring for me between the time I was relinquished and adopted. My adoption was through a county agency in the State of California. I've always known I was adopted. I was raised with an adoptive brother who was a few years older than me. We have been fully estranged for many years. Both of my adoptive parents have passed away. My adoption would be considered a success story. I was raised in a good home with good parents. I loved my adoptive parents and miss them dearly. Still, I felt out of place and thought of my birth mother every single day for as long as I can remember. Adoption was rarely spoken about in our home and it was made clear that we were not to ask questions.

I searched for over 20 years before doing DNA. During that time I also conducted searches for other adoptees and was able to help many of them reunite with their families. It was extremely important to me to conduct my own search. I wanted to be the one to find my family and make contact personally. A year after doing my own DNA test I found my entire birth family within a two week period.

I found my birth father, who had no knowledge of me, but was thrilled I found him. We had a wonderful relationship until his passing two years after we met. I miss him so much. I am still in contact with his wife who was the love of his life. I also found and am in full reunion with my maternal half sister. We are extremely close. My oldest daughter and her share the same first name. I've met and am in reunion with two paternal half sisters. I also met my paternal half brother at our fathers funeral but he has no desire to have a relationship. I'm also in reunion with my paternal uncle, aunts, several cousins, and extended family. I still have relationships with my adoptive aunts and a few cousins.

Had my mother used her true name I would have found her 20 years sooner, although it's doubtful she would have been able to leave the hospital with me. Sadly, she had passed away four years before I ever began searching. I still think of her daily and miss her horribly. Other than my sister, I have no contact, nor have I reunited with any other maternal family.

I decided to write using my birth name. I coincidentally share my first and middle birth names with my adoptive mother, although with different spellings.

Due to the laws in the State of California I am unable to have access to my Original Birth Certificate. Currently only 10 states allow Adoptees to access their Original Birth Certificate. Please ask your state lawmakers to change this law.

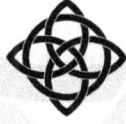

JANE ELLEN SLIWKA
(NATALIE ANNE PETTIGREW)
BRISBANE, AUSTRALIA

The Flourish Experience

IT HAS BEEN MIND BLOWING, going back through my notes from a whole year of Flourish classes and dissecting how the learnings that I gained intersected with my life over the last year. I've had many hard years in my life, and 2021 was up there as one of the most challenging. How I came to learn about Flourish is a story in and of itself. I had been working as a Post Adoption Practitioner for a small non-government organisation in Brisbane, Queensland, Australia. I have degrees in both Social Work and Psychology. In 2020 a former colleague and I started an adoption podcast from the perspective of mothers and fathers who had lost a child to adoption, adopted people and others such as authors, activists, politicians, researchers and professionals who are informed about the adoption experience. My former colleague had interviewed Pam Cordano about her book *10 Foundations for a Meaningful Life* which we had initially heard about through the *Adoptees On* podcast, hosted by Haley Radke. As a result, I met Pam for the first time in a Zoom meeting to discuss the podcast interview. I hadn't read her book at that point, but did a quick search and felt an immediate affinity with Pam. Her book is dedicated to Viktor Frankl, the Holocaust survivor and creater of logotherapy, a form of existential therapy. I had read this book at the age of 20 as a part of my psychology degree and it had a profound impact on me, particularly as I saw parallels with the adoption experience. When I heard that Pam was co-facilitating Flourish with her friend Anne Heffron, I immediately signed up to attend. It was exactly what I knew that I'd needed in my life for a long time. Working in adoption, supporting others with their adoption experience for the past eight years was taking a toll, - especially since I hadn't found somebody capable of supporting me in my own adoptee experience or an appropriate professional supervisor.

One of the best things about Flourish was that it wasn't all serious. There were so many moments of laughter. My favourite example, related to a prompt that Anne and Pam asked us to write about just a couple of days before my 34th birthday. It went something like this: "Imagine you are in full ownership of your life. You're in your car —who is in the car with you? What three things do you throw out the window and what song is playing?" I decided that I was throwing out the notion that I have to prove my worth to others, instead of embodying the fact that I am inherently worthy. I also wanted to throw out all the people who didn't have my best interests at heart or who saw me as a threat or competition. The third thing that I wanted to throw out was a lack of self-care.

Pam then asked me to think about this a little and draw on magic if I wanted. She asked me: "How would you identify the people who aren't for you?" I said "Well, there is a big sign that ejects from the roof of my car when I pull a lever. The lever gets pulled when I encounter somebody who doesn't seem to have my best interests at heart (code for: I express my needs and they don't listen/can't meet me). The sign simply says "Fuck you." It's a warning if you like. If they don't take notice of the sign and change their course, another lever causes a big arm to come out. This scoops them up and deposits them in a swamp, away from me, where they can figure their shit out for themselves." A little harsh, perhaps... But an important shift for an adoptee who had become very good at serving others and their needs. Plus, at least I wasn't saying I was going to run them down in my car!!! Unbeknownst to me at the time I shared with this the Flourish class through my laughter, this was exactly how the rest of my year would play out and in the end, it wouldn't turn out to be so funny after all.

One of my greatest realisations as a result of being a part of Flourish was that my involvement in the world-wide adoption community is far deeper and greater than any organisation that I may work for. I will always be doing this work in one way or another for the rest of my life. When I lost respect for the organisation that I was working for and felt devalued, emotionally unsafe and helpless, with the presence and support of the Flourish Community (and others in my life), I was able to put all of my cards on the table and ultimately decide that what they were offering me in both an emotional and practical sense simply wasn't good enough. When presented with another opportunity, I decided 'I deserve better.' This is not an easy realisation for an adoptee to come to. And the realisation was only the first part of a deeply painful process in leaving the organisation and more importantly the people who had felt like my family for the past five years. The reactions to my decision were also soul-destroying. This led me to 'The Nothing Place' (Pam dubbed this as a place adoptees go that feels like death). I felt rage, despair and moments I couldn't go on in my new role as the Team Leader of another adoption support organisation. I didn't feel that I had the energy to 'give' anything to anyone. I also felt the enormous loss of the podcast that was so important to me in regards to raising awareness of adoption issues on a global scale, as well as other projects I had been intensely passionate about and cared deeply for.

Partly as a result of Flourish, I had developed a mantra early in 2021: 'choose people who choose you.' This was a big call for an adoptee, who for many years would have vomited at the rhetoric about adoptees being 'chosen' (and still would). I had felt for my entire childhood that I just needed to 'get back to' my birth mother (who hadn't chosen me) and distance myself from my adoptive parents who were giving me their all and living with every bit of distance that I was putting in their way for years on end. They even supported me throughout my reunion, hosted events with my birth family present and supported my choice to work within the field of adoption. I realise now that they did choose me in a very real and authentic sense through these acts of support.

About half way through the year, the Flourish group started referring to one another as our 'Flourish Family.' Pam and Anne had outlined at the beginning of the year that Flourish is a family where you don't have to forsake parts of yourself in order to belong to the group. Also, a very big statement for a group of adoptees, who from the beginning of life have had to try to 'fit in' to ensure our survival. I believe that it was being a part of this community that enabled me to take the risk of 'losing' my work family. Feeling a part of something true and real, helped me to be able to make brave choices with my life and risk the aloneness that this may bring. It also helped me to learn who my 'real' family is, in the process. I didn't have the benefit of meeting up with other flourish members (with the exception of one), due to living in Australia during a global pandemic!! But I did learn more about the people already in my life and who to bring in closer as my chosen family.

In a moment of pain and despair, soon after leaving my job, I reached out to my long-term friend, Bethany. As I sat on her couch, sobbing into my hands, she verbalised everything that I needed to hear in that moment. Without any prior knowledge, she even alluded to things that had been discussed in our Flourish classes. That is how well she has come to know me over the years. She said "You are not 'too much.' Anybody who thinks that does not deserve you. You are allowed to want and need family. We are your family," referring to herself, her husband and her son - my godson. Other people 'stepped up' at this time also. These are the people who I now know that I want and need in my life moving forward. We need to empower ourselves and each other as adoptees to make these choices and to even remember that we have these choices now as adults. Often we can feel as though we are begging to belong (sometimes in places that aren't healthy for us). Yet, our time on this earth is limited and so is our energy. When we let go of 'false family, 'a concept discussed in Flourish, we have more to give to those who we choose and who choose us.

I think it's also important to remember that things are rarely black and white. In a moment when I felt completely abandoned and discarded by every person who had felt like my family previously, I simply didn't know how to go on ... So, I phoned my birth mother in a moment of complete despair and told her "I'm really not ok and I don't know what to do." She said "I'm glad you called me. I've always wanted to be your mother but I have felt you haven't wanted me in that role." And it's true ... Earlier in 2021, Pam Cordano had said in a Flourish class "The universe rewards the truth." This gave me the strength to tell my birth mother that her excessive alcohol consumption makes me feel unsafe and necessitates limits in our relationship. This remains a painful and complicated truth. However, it has been a relief to say it to her for the first time after 17 years of reunion. Despite how hard this would have been for her to hear, the fact that a couple of months later she could be there for me in that moment of pain and anguish is probably something I'll remember for the rest of my life.

In another Flourish class full of laughter, we were asked to 'grade our parents' and provide a rationale for the grades we choose. I surprised myself by saying about my birth father (who I always saw as 'the good guy') "loving me and caring on some level isn't enough. You have to show it. You have to take action. I deserve more than passive caring." It all hit me like a ton of bricks that the romantic interest I'd been pursuing pointlessly for four years, had recently echoed the same sentiments as my birth father (in a letter that my birth father wrote just after my birth) where he said "It would have been too hard to keep you." I shared this with my birth mother not long after I had the realisation and she immediately burst into tears and said, "That's exactly it. Everything is just 'too hard' for him." And she apologised. She apologised for choosing him over me, all those years ago.

In Flourish we talked about 'mutuality' and 'bonding.' We were reminded that as babies we cried and cried and our mother never came back. We never knew what it felt like to cry and actually experience our mother soothing us and helping us to settle. We learned that in order to survive we needed to meet the need of the other. My adoptive parents had a need for a "perfect" child. My Grandma would tell me, shaking her head, that my Dad wanted nothing less than a perfect child and would discipline me accordingly. I realised that maybe I became a Social Worker because I was programmed from an early age to meet the needs of others. Yet, I'd now reached a point of burnout and felt that I couldn't do it anymore. When I started my new job, amidst my grief and heartbreak, I was told how happy everybody was to have me there as their team leader and my manager said how excited she was (presumably regarding what I could do for the service). I told her on my first day, sitting across from her, "I know you're excited, but I'm not." Who says that to a new manager, at a new job? Apparently I do, perhaps aided by the realness and authenticity that I had come to know through Flourish. It didn't take me long to work out what was going on here ... This is what I would have liked to have told my adoptive mother as an infant the day she brought me home. I would have wanted to tell her that whilst her needs were being met, all I wanted was for her to take me back to my birth family and for them to do whatever it would take to keep me. We were reminded in Flourish that we couldn't speak then, but we can now. We have the ability to 'take action' when we need to and in many ways our life depends on it.

In the weeks that followed I verbalised my grief, pain and the feeling that I didn't believe that I could continue in this job. And what happened next blew me away. She choose me. My manager encouraged me to do what was best for me, but to take time and think about it. When I started asking about what she needed and what the organisation needed and how sorry I was, she didn't entertain those questions for a moment. Instead, she asked me what I needed. When I said "Well, I do feel calmer when I speak to you..." she smiled and suggested that we meet more regularly. This has enabled me to continue in the job and it really has been incredibly soothing, comforting and empowering. As I write this, I am reminded of the flourish prompt that asked us to consider what it would take to turn away from 'false family' and toward a family that 'feels real'.

So, when I look back on 2021, there was a lot lost and a lot gained. Growth is not easy but it's a bit easier when you have a community (family) by your side who knows the same pain and who is similarly focussed on healing and authenticity. I know that I will remain in contact with many of the other Flourishers and I can only hope that when the world opens up, I will meet more of them in person.

I am also reminded of Pam's comment that adoptee healing is non-linear... Just when you think you're getting somewhere, you wind up back in the same loop. So, my other hope is that each time we find ourselves in The Nothing Place, we're a little stronger than last time and a little better at getting ourselves (and each other) out of there and back in the world making choices, living our best lives and changing the world. And when it comes to changing the world, I'm reminded that sometimes there can be a lot of pain and uncertainty to get through first, before we start to see the 'payoff' for our courage and truth telling. Yet, I've seen the pay-off before. So, for any adoptee who is struggling (including myself), hang in there.

JANE'S STORY:

Jane's story: I was born in 1987 and named Natalie Anne by my birth parents. I stayed with them in the hospital for a week after my birth. Other family members came to visit and we have photos together. I then went to a foster home for 10 weeks, prior to my adoptive parents picking me up and my adoption being finalised. My adoptive parents named me Jane Ellen and the adoption was facilitated by the Queensland Government in Australia. I was raised as an only child and don't remember being told that I was adopted (I recall always knowing). However, there was a lot of silence around the topic of adoption and I felt very alone with my feelings. When I was 18 years old, I reunited with my birth parents, who had gone on to marry each other, and met my brother (then 11 years old) and my sister (10 years old at the time). I am still in contact with my birth family and see them several times a year. This has been a roller coaster ride for sure and continues to be. My adoptive father died when I was 26 years old and five months later, my adoptive mother died when I was 27 years old. As I sat on my Dad's hospital room floor, as he was dying, I was simultaneously writing a job application for a position in post-adoption support. He told me 'I really hope you get it Jane'. By the time I was successful in obtaining the position, he had died. I have been working in the field since 2013, first as a practitioner and now as a Team Leader. In Australia, there are Government funded support services that assist adoptees and their relatives to search for and reunite with one another, in addition to counseling and group support. I am proud to assist adoptees and their families to heal and to have been a co-founder and co-host of a podcast to support education and healing on a larger scale. I am thankful to Pam, Anne and the Flourish Community for showing me that there are so many meaningful ways of contributing to the world-wide adoption community.

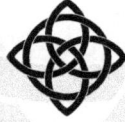

JENNIFER JAMES
ARIZONA

AS A LITTLE GIRL, I wondered why my adoptive parents' names replaced the names of my biological parents on my legal birth certificate. This document is about me, yet it is not true. *I was not born from this woman and man who adopted me. Who are the people who created me? Why is "it" a secret? What is so bad about my birth that caused its details to be legally changed? Why are my records in Santa Fe? Why can't I have access to them? Where do I come from?*

I did not know I had Hispanic origins until my 18th birthday, when my adoptive parents gave me a brief resume about my biological parents:

The Way I Look On Paper

Biological Mother:	Biological Father:	Me:
• Spanish-Anglo	• English-Irish	• Hispanic & Caucasian
• Catholic	• Lutheran	• Non Denominational
• "around 19 years old"	• "in his late 20's"	• 'late 40's"
• 5'3" tall	• 6'4" tall	• 5'9" tall
• Brown hair	• Blonde hair	• Prematurely grey hair
• Brown eyes	• Blue eyes	• Light brown eyes.

Some people say I look Hispanic, others say they can't see *"it"*. I feel invisible when they can't see *"it"* even though I don't even know what *"it"* means.

Adoption ... God's Answer To Everyone's Prayer

My adoptive parent's profile fit all the boxes: They were educated, healthy and financially stable, yet unable to achieve a family "the natural way" after almost ten years of marriage. My adoptive mother had been through three miscarriages, and her obstetrician/gynocologist had a young patient about to give birth to a child she was planning to relinquish – that child is me.

The doctor aligned his patient with an attorney, who arranged a closed private adoption between the attorney, my adoptive parents and my biological mother. My adoptive parents' finances would cover my biological mother's living and medical expenses. My adoption could not have been more planned or more perfect. *Or could "it"?*

My birth was the answer to so many people's prayers! My adoptive parents yearned for children. My biological mother, an unmarried teenager, was most likely encouraged to relinquish her child. My biological father did not participate in any of the details of my placement, which is what I'm told he wanted. The love, prayers and saviorship of my adoptive parents' church family supported my birth plan. My birth was announced at the pulpit that Sunday morning for all to hear! God brought a child to their church for them to rear. Closed adoption also aligned with the American medical and legal practices of the times. My severance from my biological family at two-days old was legal, socially acceptable, justifiable, prayed for, and even celebrated. Everyone believed that the baby would not know the difference.

Just six months after I was adopted, my adoptive mother gave birth to their own biological child. She had been three months pregnant when they signed the papers and brought me home. Within six months, this childless wedded couple had become a fruitful family of four, with two daughters a mere six months apart in age.

There are many people who insist that everyone has had my best interest at heart. That I was a miracle and so lucky to have been adopted. That I've had *"it"* so much better than so many other children in this world and should be grateful. How on earth could I have an ungrateful bone in my body? From the outside, my life looks like an adoption fairytale, and many would say I have had the most *gifted* of lives.

I feel guilty and ashamed for saying this but why is there a hole in my heart? Why can't I just be happy? Can anyone grasp my feelings of isolation, being alone, and surviving?

The Baby Knows the Difference

There are no pictures of me before I was two days old. The first picture is one of me being handed to my adoptive parents as if I were a present, or a "gift" as I, and many adoptees, are often labeled.

My adoptive parents were told that my biological mother had a very difficult time handing me over at the hospital that day. I wonder when my 6 pound 3 ounce body realized that I had been separated from her for the last time? At some point I had to begin to interpret my safety. I must have cried for as long as my body would tolerate. Did I do this often or only a few times until I eventually realized my reality?

My New Normal: *I was on my own never to see my biological mother again.*

Ever since I can remember, I have craved connection and a desire to "fit in." Not like being one of the popular kids at school, but as if my life depended on it. Sheer survival and fear of death. My craving for connection is primal.

If my life were an experiment of survival, the litmus test would be my constant flexing, stretching and shrinking to achieve homeostasis in the safety and security of my environment. *If she could leave me, anyone can!* The boundaries I hold are rigid, keep me safe, and allow for me to take care of myself first. Adopted also means adapted. Adoptees adapt because we are mammals wanting our mothers. We must feed, we need touch, we need her sound and vibration. I wanted nourishment, I wanted her warm touch, her verbal soothing, and the maternal skin to skin intimacy only a mother and child know. At some moment I crossed a tipping point realizing I would never feel her heartbeat, hear her tummy gurgle, listen to her sweet calming voice, feel her pulse, smell her chemical pheromones, embrace her touch outside of the womb, or feel the warmth and safety of her body temperature again. At some point I had to unclench and give up in defeat with the dysregulation of knowing I had been relinquished by my biological creator. Every nonverbal and verbal communication technique I used would be for survival because my life depended on it. My undeveloped, preverbal brain knew it. Her smell was gone. Her voice was gone. Her taste was gone. Her touch was gone. I could no longer see her.

As I gained understanding, I couldn't wrap my tiny brain around how my biological mother's relinquishment of me also fit into the same category as "miracle."

Who would pray for such a horrible thing to happen?

Everyone was *happy* that my sister had her biological mother; "our mother".

Why were they not *sad* in knowing that I did not have my biological mother?

Why am I the only one crying? Why are strangers taking care of me? Nothing smells the same. Nothing sounds the same. I want my mommy!

Becoming a Mother Changed Everything

On the day I learned I was pregnant with my own child, my perception of my adoption changed. I was now going to bear my own child and live through a life experience I knew my biological mother had endured. I was holding a part of her inside of me. I eagerly awaited to meet the first person in the world known to me as a genetic relative. Getting to know my daughter from the womb to human was not a process I could have interrupted. In my own experience, I cannot understand how a mother could give away her child. Enduring pregnancy with no matriarchal family members to ask about their pregnancies made the experience extra frightening and lonely. I leaned on medical professionals anxiously asking questions about every symptom. My job became to constantly maintain her and my safety...*surviving.*

I would not have known my birth mother had complications during my birth until I, too, experienced many of my own requiring extra hospitalization both during and post partum. The stress caused my adoptive parents to recall a memory shortly after my birth when they were asked by the attorney if they would be willing to pay for additional days of hospitalization and medical expenses for my biological mother due to complications from her pregnancy. I oddly felt a deep level of connection with my biological mother while I sat in the hospital alone throughout my pregnancy. I wondered if she was alone during her labor and delivery with me. The outcome from the complications of my high-risk pregnancy meant I would only become a biological mother once in my lifetime. *Was I also my biological mother's only pregnancy?*

And yes, because I too had the question and needed to be sure: my biological mother's medical expenses were loyally covered with no pushback from my adoptive parents.

Family

I gave *The Primal Wound* by Nancy Verrier to each of my adoptive parents for Christmas in 2020 while in Flourish. The book is a permanent fixture on many adoptee's bookshelves. Nancy does a beautiful job of uniting perspectives of communication between the triad of adoption (adoptee, adoptive parents, biological parents).

My adoptive mother finished reading the book in one sitting, and immediately called me. She confessed that my pediatrician prescribed phenobarbital to help us cope with my cries when I was an infant. She told me she now felt horrible about it, and wished she could change what happened, but wanted me to know the facts. Her honesty and vulnerability in sharing her truth showed me that she and my adoptive father were doing their best back then with the information they had. Their need to seek medication to calm me also validated that they saw my struggle through my cries. I oddly felt seen, soothed, and nurtured when she told me she resorted to medication to ease my pain. Being a mother myself I might have sought the same treatment for my daughter had she been inconsolable. Nobody is perfect and people with the best of intentions make mistakes. My adoptive mom's willingness to read a book so important to me in one sitting so soon after I gave it to her was priceless. We have always done the work to preserve our mother-daughter relationship and pursue new depths. I believe we crossed a new bridge of safety that day.

My adoptive father is no different. I have watched him weep for me and open his mind to my perspective about my circumstances without judgment to attempt to understand my perspective as best as he can. I believe he would do anything he could to ease my pain, yet wisely knows he can do nothing but patiently let me do my own healing work.. What I need is not something an adoptive parent can give a child no matter how much love and support they provide us.

My adoptive parents have more than fulfilled their legal commitment to my adoption contract. They have never stopped unconditionally loving me without abandon as I have learned to endure the complex reality of my circumstances. They have also given me every therapeutic tool I've ever asked for to help save myself. I am finally able to see my adoptive parents' truth from a new human perspective and can connect my years of testing them to my abandonment fears. *Please don't be mad at me for appearing ungrateful.*

Adoptive families are not prepared to field common questions from curious family and friends within earshot of the adoptee.

"Now which one is the adopted one again?" Was a common question my adoptive parents were routinely asked as we grew up changing before family and friend's eyes. I have no doubt that the question came from honest intentions, however the micro aggressions I experienced felt objectifying and often became unbearable.

My sister and I have always had a tight connection. I can pick on her but I'll kick your ass if you even try to co-conspire with me because I would protect her with my life. We have had World War III a hundred times over and always reunite over happy hour or celebratory dinner. We couldn't survive without each other and literally communicate using a nonverbal "twin like" secret language. We were the ultimate nature vs. nurture experiment growing up, and I sometimes still feel like we are today. Those who know us have always been curious about which of our behaviors/traits are genetic or environmental. No matter how my adoptive parents attempted to combat competition or silence other's need to share their opinions and comparisons about our similarities and differences, people's verbal vomit happened. My sister also quickly learned that my adoption was a sensitive subject for me so if she wanted to tease me, it was at the top of her playlist to attempt to trigger my tears knowing it would ignite immediate embarrassment for me. What we also didn't know when my sister and I were growing up is that her behaviors and communication struggles would have put her on today's diagnostic scale of high functioning autism. Her behaviors were often out of her span of impulse control and therefore created an added family dynamic for our parents to manage that my sister remembers very little of yet I hold vivid multiple traumatic memories because I did not know how to interpret her actions towards me. I use the example because I believe many families are not adequately prepared to field questions from siblings or outsiders about their family adoption story. Lack of preparedness can lead to constant objectification of the adoptee and cause permanent complex trauma. *I hate being adopted!*

Adoptees struggle with relationships because we don't understand them after such a primal wound. When I was talking to Nancy Verrier earlier this year on the phone, she said that everyone should watch *Animal Planet* more closely and frequently. "You all," (this is how Nancy refers to adoptees) "You all did not deserve to be separated from your mothers." She went on to tell me about how she had memories from growing up on a farm when an animal would lose its mother during birth, she explained, it was very infrequent that her family could get the animal to bond to a "new" adoptive mother and therefore the baby animal would fail to thrive and die. She remembered as a little girl feeling so sad when seeing this unnatural placement fail. In our conversation, she said "It just isn't natural". Nancy helped me understand how important it is to incorporate biological family into the upbringing of an adoptee or person in a guardianship situation. She also encouraged me to initiate my reunion and told me about all of the biological mothers she has worked with and their desire to know we as adoptees are ok. I will be forever grateful for this conversation with her and her work for the adoptee community.

My adoptive parents divorced when I was 21. I took it hard. I felt like their part of the adoption deal fell through. *Where was the stability I had been promised?* I wouldn't understand until going through a divorce of my own years later just how complex life can get.

Flourish helped me find my voice within my adoptive family to talk about my adoption without filtering my feelings in an attempt to protect other's feelings. Flourish fueled my courage to ask questions. I am in the minority of Flourish members who have living adoptive parents willing to answer their adoption questions. Since Flourish, I have had multiple in-depth conversations with my adoptive parents, step parents, and sister. They all continue to be nothing but supportive of me beginning my search *when I am ready.*

I have relied on pure honesty and authenticity in these conversations. Even when it hurts. Even when we don't like what we see in each other. Sometimes the discomfort of our conversation slices so thin and deep that I want to run. My fear of abandonment is always just under the surface ready to activate. I tread water to protect my adoptive family relationships because of all they have done for me, but now also work to save myself. The shift in my conversations with others about my adoption is that I can now protect myself first. I still experience the flood of negative body sensations as they race into every cell taking me back to a preverbal unsafe place when I ask a difficult question. The difference is, I can now observe and identify my feelings of abandonment to regulate myself and remember that *I am safe and they are not going to leave me.*

My yearning to search and initiate reunion with my biological family comes and goes. I believe that it has been hard to begin this search because my adoptive family and extended family have always been so fruitful. I have been showered with parents throughout my life. Not only do I have my adoptive parents, but their amazing spouses, who have been in my life for more than 25 years each. I also maintain relationships with my ex-husband, and his two sets of parents which brings my total to four pairs of "parents" (adoptive, step, and in-laws). I had amazing god-parents, and have played the "adopted" child in many friends' families over the years. All of my parents and influencers have supported me throughout different parts of my life showing me that love and support are plentiful and will always be there in good times and bad. *Why do I still feel so disconnected and alone? Why can't I just be "happy"?*

Depression and Mental Health

At age 16, I was diagnosed with depression. I was seen by the top professionals in our city and my adoptive parents were told that it was something chemical in my brain and something I could not help. The diagnosis oddly validated my feelings of being "different" from my adoptive family and even gave me an excuse to hate my own DNA. It also gave me permission to question my existence and wonder what was inherently wrong with me. *Why was I given up for adoption?* My patterns of rebellion grew. Would these pills really help me feel *"better"* and get through *"it"*? *Whatever "it"* was.

Once the medical community quantified my maladaptive coping techniques and behaviors into a tidy list of mental health symptoms a diagnosis could be made. I had a new identity and another level of experts for my family and me to consult to figure *"it"* out. *Am I the problem? Do others in my biological family also struggle with depression or other mental health illnesses?*

The depression I experience as an adoptee is often unexplainable to others. As an adult, I still feel infantilized by my loved ones because their scope of judging an adoptee's happiness is focused on what adoptees have been *given* or were *saved* from, not the grief we experience from losing our biological family.

I learned at a very young age to be grateful for my adoption. Women would pull me aside at church and tell me how lucky I was to be adopted and to always be a "good little girl". Those women were right, I was lucky, and I tried to be good and appear grateful. I also learned that the world did not have space to hear about my pain surrounding my relinquishment. It was so painful to them that they could not possibly discuss it with me. In fact, much of the world cannot stand to see anything other than the beauty in an adoption story. This is how the adoptee becomes silenced under layer upon layer of toxic positivity. Nobody wants to think that the prayer of a beautiful adoption story also means the shattering of a biological mother's story. The scarlet letter of shame placed on her is not the happily ever after comfortable story of adoption. The duality of my gratitude and need to protect everyone who had saved me combined with my pain from being relinquished eventually silenced me. No matter what I tried to say to express my pain, it was trumped by what I had already been given as the *next best option* for someone in my circumstances, and therefore I needed to learn to be grateful.

Depression is a journey. I still fight it. The frequency and intensity are unpredictable. Through the years, I have collected additional diagnoses from the medical community to help them quantify the way I cope from my relinquishment and adoption. Their coding has allowed me to be able to save my own life, maintain a full time job, and build my own tool belt through therapy and treatment when the need arises.

My experience with mental health care and self care is like that of a car. Sometimes I need to go in for several days of repair and retreat, and sometimes just a tune up and regular maintenance can keep me balanced. I have had the same psychiatrist for over 15 years and the same therapist for over 5. They have fought for me and watched me fight for myself.

When I am feeling healthy, the last thing I want to do is initiate a reunion with my biological family. I find adoption to be a burden and statistically know that reunion will add new complications and dynamics to my life once I initiate contact. I tell my doctor and therapy team, "Why would I want to make things messy?" Then we re-group and discuss the elephant in the room. Reunion is the one thing I have not attempted in order to heal my depression, anxiety, eating disorder, OCD, and trauma (I told you there was a list!).

My parents, sister, family, friends, and team know that when I am not well, I yearn to know my medical background and story. They want me to have the answers but never push me because they know how highly sensitive I am to feelings of abandonment. I will forever be grateful to them for letting me keep my own pace, even though we have all discussed my risk of possibly never meeting my biological family if I don't take action. I witness how hard it is for them to unconditionally love me yet respect my boundary about the pace of my reunion. I feel so seen and loved when they give me the time and space I need to process my feelings about reunion.

Reunion with my biological family is simply the one thing I have resisted doing. As of yet, there is no storm I haven't survived, with the tribe I was given. My adoptive family tree is layered with unconditional love and support as was planned and prior to my birth. These are the reasons I have not reached out to anyone in my biological family ... *and the fact that I fear rejection.*

Being Adopted is Expensive

I have spent more than 30 years in therapy learning about myself while the medical community has categorized my behaviors and symptoms. There is no line item or ICD9 code for *"being adopted"* yet we are over represented in both the mental health and prison systems. We are also 25 percent more likely to attempt suicide. These are epidemic public health numbers and had I not had the support of my family, friends, medical team, and employer, I would not have survived.

I bring up the expense of adoption because acceptance of my circumstances with professional help has been costly in many areas of my life. Financially, I have spent and continue to spend a lot of money on my mental healthcare. My appointments, groups, and therapies also take time away from living my life and enjoying my relationships to their fullest. I have spent so much time tending to this feeling that I am not enough. Broken. Unfinished.

I joined Flourish after I had been participating in a three-day a week online Eating Disorder Intensive Outpatient meal support group during the pandemic. I experienced multiple relapses in my eating disorder after a divorce in 2014, a breast cancer diagnosis in 2015 and the pandemic in 2020. By the fall of 2020, my eating disorder was stable and I no longer had the need for multiple days of group work and meal support. In a past life I would have celebrated this accomplishment, but this time I was scared. I still had a need for connection with other people like me. Throughout this relapse I met several people in my programs who had eating disorders and were also adopted. At one point 50% of my eating disorder group was composed of adoptees. I was uncovering so many parallels and felt like I was on to something. If healing in a virtual group environment worked so well for my eating disorder and other symptoms, I had hope. Flourish became the perfect solution to safely step down from my eating disorder group and also fill my need for weekly community support and to finally meet and talk to other adoptees.

Flourish was also not free. I was now choosing to invest money in myself without a co-pay or a doctor's order to try and soothe my yearning to get over my deepest fears surrounding my adoption. It turned out to be the best money I ever spent on myself. I joke with my writing coach, Anne Heffron, about the constant expense of adoption and that she is part of that when I pay her monthly fee. A price that is more than worth it. I need her because she "gets it." I secured her as a coach before Flourish ended to not only continue my work but also to selfishly keep myself supported in an adoptee writing community. I have no intention of stopping my work with her because I need her skillset. She taught me the concept that adoptees need adoptees. The questions she encourages us to answer for ourselves, no matter how uncomfortable, are necessary in healing. We have lost years of our lives NOT talking about adoption. Our voices matter.

I have learned expensive lessons, lost precious time, and carried the shame of my adoption without knowing what to do with *"it"* while also watching everyone who loves me try to solve *"it"* for me. The survival of an adoptee requires money, time, unconditional love, and extreme patience from others and the self. Sadly the stars do not align for all adoptees and we lose many to suicide.

Discussing the burden and shame of adoption makes me think of the words from the women at church who used to remind me of my need to always be grateful for my adoption. My practice of gratitude routinely turned into guilt for circumstances I had no control over.

Flourish allowed me to buy a gift for myself. Something I didn't even know was for sale. Agency. A life that no longer makes me feel like I am a list of diagnoses or a cost to another person. I am different and changed after 16 months of writing weekly in an adoptee community. The words that flow out of me are authentic and are my truth. I have had the freedom to write without judgment about the radical topic of adoption and my experience as an adoptee. Before finding this connection, I often felt "told" how to feel. I have let go of other's visions for myself and am gaining back control of my life.

Ancestry

After starting Flourish I bought both Ancestry and 23andMe kits. For a long time, I had both unopened boxes physically collecting dust on my desk and mentally creating a shame game that was riddling me with guilt, fear and anxiety. I am a fucking breast cancer survivor. Why can't I do this?

Reunion has always felt like accomplishing the un-accomplishable. I wanted the courage I saw in my Flourish peers who had walked the path of reunion before me. Their warrior energy helped me to take my DNA tests and mail them in.

I received my results in the spring of 2021. They validated the non-identifying information I obtained from New Mexico and also gave me the missing links to acquire obituaries on my maternal and paternal sides and locate my biological family. In a matter of hours I found *her* photo on Facebook. The mirroring is incredible. She looks safe and healthy. She has long grey hair like me. Seeing her immediately puts my mind at ease. As for my biological father, I have not found *him* yet. I have located his sister, my paternal aunt. He is one of her two brothers. *I wonder if he will be mad when he finds out.*

It has been over a year since I published my contact information and photograph on ancestry.com and 23andMe. I have been matched to three biological close family members: a maternal aunt, a maternal uncle, and a paternal aunt. I also have 4 first cousins, twenty five second cousins and 167 third cousins. I have yet to hear from or meet any of them. Who is waiting for who? When is the time right? What life event will it take for one of us to reach out? I am no longer a secret.

JENNIFER'S STORY:

I am a female adoptee born in the mid 1970's in Albuquerque, New Mexico. For the first two days of my life I was identified in the hospital as "Unknown Baby Girl" until I was relinquished by my biological mother and taken home at two days old by my adoptive parents. I am told my biological mother had a very difficult time letting me go. To this day, my birth record is sealed in Santa Fe to protect the identities of my biological parents. I've had my birth file opened, acquired all non-identifying information, and maintained my current contact information in case my biological parents ever want to get in touch with me. Reunion is a switch that neither I or my biological family have flipped.

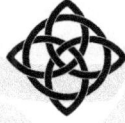

JULIA RICHARDSON

UNITED KINGDOM

The Nothing Place

THE LAST TWO WEEKS I have been in my 'nothing place.' When Pam Cordano started to talk about the 'nothing place' I knew immediately what she meant and I knew that it was where I was. We all knew what she meant. All the adoptees in our Flourish class. We knew. We felt it, we understood. It is our place. For some of us it is terrifying, for some of us it is a safe space, for all of us it is familiar and a place where we are familiar but where we know we are strangers in a strange land. We are the aliens in the other world, the Muggle world, the civilian non-adopted world. Right here in this space in my world, in my home, in my body, in my relationships and in my everyday life I have been living in my nothing place.

This is my nothing place. I am tired of trying. This week I gave up and gave in. I ate all the food I don't usually eat. I can't fill myself because there isn't enough and I am empty. I can't say it. I can't talk about it. It takes too much energy. I just have to be here in it. I know I have to go through it. 'It' is the nothing place. Even now, at 63 years of age, I am the overwhelming whole body hungry baby. I continue to feel abandoned and starving and the wrong person is trying to feed me with the wrong food. Now, most often, that person is me. My hunger feels like a shame-filled greed – impossible to satisfy. I am tired of adapting and explaining and being compliant.

What happens when I eat all the food? I am eating until I stop and then I can be where I am.

The nothing place makes me feel afraid because I thought I was connected even just a little bit but now I know I wasn't. The connection was so tenuous and it wasn't even real. My birth family members don't understand me and they are now hostile and I feel like I am grounded in nothingness where I am rejected and abandoned and disappointed and lost and dying from being unseen and unknown. I have been eating because I know that place and I know how to do that. I also know that I will stop. This hunger will not consume me totally unless I allow it to. Maybe for a while being consumed and eaten alive is what I want because I want to disappear.

I have someone who is mine and who sees me but she is not adopted so the nothing place is not hers. She can see me in here but she can't be in here with me. I didn't know that until today.

I feel as if I am floating away from shore. It is easier to lie back and float and watch the sky and go with the currents and be taken away. The water is cold but it carries me and I don't have to fight it. Part of me is scared of the hunger and the floating because they are unstoppable and monumental and part of me, the core of me, knows somehow she is safe because I am floating into the nothingness. It is inside and outside me, I am nothingness. The image of my adoptee tribe floating here in nothingness with me is like being born into a family where I am known. We are part of the same nothing place. This is our country. We have our own language. Nothing is where we are when we are born and taken away from our universe. Our mother is our universe before we are born and she is all there is and all we have when we slide into the world. And then our universe is taken away so where are we? We are nothing. There is no comparative experience than that of a baby that has lost its mother. That baby has lost its whole universe. Attachment theory has all been written and understood from the perspective of someone who has a universe. From the position of being a human being with a mother. This is not our experience. We are always ultimately motherless. Don't argue with me about this. I don't need your opinion because I know that this is the reality of those of us who have lived it.

Yes this is a freedom I haven't experienced before. I knew that I was crawling towards something big over the last two weeks. I have skinned my hands and knees and eaten my body weight in comfort food but now I have stopped. I am enough. I don't need to consume myself any more. I am consumed by nothingness for I am she and she is me. We are one. I am floating in the other-world place because I know who I am and where I am and there is no longer any need to explain. My tribe is floating here with me so I am never ever alone any more.

"Are You Anti-Adoption?"

Today someone sent me this message in response to something I had posted on social media about adoption being a trauma. This was my reply:

I'm adopted. I am not totally against adoption per se but I am passionate about developing understanding of the trauma it causes for adoptees and birth mothers in particular.

I thought for a moment then I added:

P.S. With understanding and compassion adoptive parents can help their child to understand their feelings are 'normal' and that their wish to know where they have come from is also valid. There has been a conspiracy of silence, especially with closed adoption. Haha I'm on my soapbox. I just wrote a book about it, coming out soon.

He replied:

Thank you for explaining, this is helpful to understand where you are coming from.

I answered:

No worries. It's complicated.

After some reflection, I know there is so much wrong with our exchange. I fell once again into a well-worn adoptee pattern of "being nice," "making it nice" for the other person. I discounted my own views and experience and options and made them 'less than.' The truth is, I am against adoption. I hate it. I don't hate adoptive parents. I hope adoptive parents will read this. But adoption itself? Honestly, it sucks. It is a legalised method of severing babies and children from the people they are genetically connected to. Adoption takes away a person's rights to their identity. Adoption strips them of living with people who look like them, think like them, feel like them. Mirroring is impossible.

My views are not popular. I have been part of the adoption system as a social worker, as a parent, as a mother of a son adopted son who was adopted by his step-father (my then- husband). And of course, as an adoptee.

I don't totally disagree with my own responses to my friend. I do know it is possible to ameliorate some of the damage done by relinquishment and severance. There are many ways in which children could be helped to not feel like millions of adult adoptees felt growing up, especially those from the closed adoption era.

We need "adoption competent" therapists. This specialty involves specific skills and knowledge around attachment and an awareness that adoption is trauma. Not sometimes. Always.

Why do adoptees have to explain? Why do I have to explain? Why do I have to justify how I feel? Why is it so shocking that my experience of adoption is such that my views about the institution are so strong? If I had been sexually abused and I said that I was anti-abuse that would be OK. I am anti-abuse and would be accepted without question. But adoption is still regarded as a 'good' thing. Adoptive parents are seen as saviours and saints, extra-special people. Most adopters adopt because of infertility. They are adopting for themselves. When we have children we do it for us not for them. And thereby hangs another thread. This is somewhere that angels fear to tread.

I am a proud member of the LGBQT and the Adoptee communities. There is incongruence to navigate there too. Gay and lesbian couples often adopt or go down other routes such as surrogacy to have a family. The child may not have any biological connection to their parents. Whose needs are being met here? There is still a severance. Severance from the Mother is a trauma for the infant, and also for the mother. This has to be understood and the trauma acknowledged, listened to and heard and allowed to exist. It is not the 'fault' of adopters that the trauma exists.

It is not the fault of the mother who relinquishes. It is not the fault of the baby who is severed. This is not a blame game but it often feels like a "no win" situation. I don't believe in the "triad" of birth parent, adopted person, adopter.

There are far more nuanced ways to look at adoption and we can no longer not ignore the huge impact that society, culture, religion, governments and institutionalized racism have on any system including how we care for or manage our children.

Food and Eating and Adoption

I was adopted as a baby. I am no longer a child but I will always be an adoptee. I have complex feelings about adoption as an institution and also about my personal experience. For a very long time I had no idea that my feelings were what you might call "normal" for someone who had been a) given away as a baby and b) lived their life in a family that wasn't theirs.

More and more people like me are clambering out of our respective closets and saying, "Here I am, this is my story, here is my voice."

Many of us have had many years of feeling silenced by a narrative that sees adoption as Just a Nice Thing. Not long ago I happened to tell someone at a social event that I was adopted. "Oh how lovely," she replied. I sort of wanted to punch her. Instead I said, "Hmm it's complicated." I expect that was the better response but some days I'm not so sure.

Another common response to saying I am adopted is, "Did you have nice parents?" Well, yes I did thank you, did you? My parents were "nice" people. But that isn't the point. Nice is not the problem. Or the solution.

I have so much to say about all this that I wrote Life In-Between, my memoir of adoption, addiction, relationships and recovery A growing number of adoptees are beginning to tell their stories on blogs and in books, in podcasts and interviews and in groups where we come together and find each other and ourselves.

In 2021 a group of adoptees committed to meet each Sunday for a whole year in a class called Flourish. The class was set up last year by Anne Heffron, author of You Don't Look Adopted, and Pam Cordano, author of 10 Foundations For a Meaningful Life. Twenty seven adoptees meeting over Zoom (thank you, Covid-19) to share our experience, to learn, grow, connect, and be together. The class isn't for therapy though it may be therapeutic. It isn't for education although I learned so much every time. We may be a self-selecting group because we recognise that adoption is a trauma and that we have been traumatised. Some of us are just making sense of our adopted lives for the first time and some of us have been working on our own healing for what feels like forever. Some of us have connected with our birth families and some have not. Some of us were rejected. Some of us found that our birth parents had died before we could meet. All our stories are different and yet … and yet … our similarities are breathtaking. We recognise each other. We understand the pain. We see each other. We listen. We cry. We laugh. We write. And after the class we talk during the week. Some of us message or speak to each other. We share what is happening in our lives and how we feel after our latest Sunday class.

Each class is intense and we all have different ways to handle how we feel afterwards. Because we are a transatlantic group, the class is early in the morning for the North Americans and in the afternoon for the Europeans. So time of a day plays a part in our comfort responses. Ron in Philadelphia goes for a walk afterwards by himself. Cat and I in the UK make dinner separately in our own homes and then eat it and watch TV. Some have a nap. Anne in California feeds the chickens and has a bike-ride. Beth is in Germany and gets back to Sunday family life. Other people are also having family time with their husbands, wives and partners and their kids or with their adoptive or birth families. Family life is always complicated.

Sometimes people are getting messages from bio-family members or other people in their lives who want or need our time and attention. And we all often have big feelings to process. Because we are quite a large group we don't all feel sad or happy, angry or heart-broken at the same time. But we can be a witness for each other and that is priceless. As adoptees we have learnt to be very good at taking care of everyone else's feelings, often before our own. We are often the observers and the mediators. We like to know what you would like to do before we can decide what we would like. We have learnt to fit in or to fit ourselves into spaces that weren't meant for our size bodies or personalities. Sometimes we feel squashed and suffocated by those spaces. Sometimes we have made ourselves so small that we hope we can get away with being invisible.

One way to manage big feelings is to soothe them away. This is a useful and important strategy otherwise known as self-care. Or is it? Sometimes self-care becomes something darker. In one of our sessions the subject of cake arose. Innocent enough you might think?

Of course it depends on your perspective. And that is what we found: It's not news that we love cake. The British sweet tooth is famous. We are the cheapskate Europeans who like chocolate in family-size packs from supermarket shelves. But sugar is a universal soother. It is so recognised now for it's pain relieving qualities that it is used medically. For some of us that is a double-edged sword.

I am someone who has had a difficult relationship with food. The connection between emotional pain and the soothing effect of food in the form of milk started before my memory begins.

When I went to my adoptive parents I was already three months old. I cried a lot. It was hard for me to settle. My new mother found that feeding me two bottles of milk instead of one sent me to sleep. I don't think it was hunger that made me cry. I had already had two homes by then and multiple "mothers" to feed me. I learnt that food and a full tummy was enough to keep me safe. I found food took the place of attachment. They became interchangeable. My hunger barometer got broken early. I don't know when I am hungry but I know when I am feeling pain that food will take it away. Not for long but for a second or two.

Both my adoptive and my birth mothers loved food,all food but especially sweets and chocolate. I had a double whammy of food confusion from nature and nurture.

Food is a primal need. Food is life. Sometimes food is love. What happens when love is food? A baby's first response is to 'root', the search of the mouth for nipple, the instinctive urge to suckle. Feeding my own babies there was the sharp intensity of a physical tug from the clamping of those hard baby gums on a nipple. A painful and pleasurable trigger that sent colostrum and then milk surging through their system and into that waiting mouth. Adopted babies often have their first feed from a bottle. We often don't know who gave us our first feed. That is my story.

Were we fed by different hands each time in the nursery or at a mother and baby home? Did foster carers get up to us at night or were we propped in our cots with a bottle?

It's well known that childhood trauma can lead to addiction. Often we think of addiction in relation to drugs and alcohol but food is addictive too, so is shopping and gambling and gaming. There are multiple ways to change how we feel.

Our group discovered a common thread of food-related experience. Cake has featured enormously in our conversations. Sharing about trauma is hard. It brings up a longing for comfort and cake is comfort on a plate. We are diverse: Black, hispanic and white. European and North American. All shapes and sizes. Male and female, although mostly female. Gay and straight. Parents and not. Siblings and not. Twins. Employed and not. Old, young and in-between.

We talked about our place at the table. What was it when we were growing up? What is our place now? Where do we belong?

Food for Thought

We had a wooden dining table that my adoptive mum was very proud of. I used to sit underneath it and play. There was a green baize tablecloth which protected the shiny surface from scratches and heat marks and the sides hung down so that when I was underneath with my crayons and paper or my dolls it felt like a cosy, safe place to make a den. One day I had a biro and I scratched my name on the underside with the pen. It felt like a dangerous, rebellion act and there was a little buzz of excitement as I saw the blue ink eat into the pale golden wood perfection of the naked wood. Mummy didn't find out until we moved house a few years later. She wasn't angry.

Food was always an issue in our house. I ate food I didn't like to be polite. Meal-times were sacred and they happened at clearly regulated intervals – the timing was sacrosanct. There were rules about what we ate and when. Certain foods were only for certain meals. Now I get a little thrill from the prospect of breakfast for dinner. Breakfast is the best meal. There are so many options in breakfast. Sweet and savoury. A 'full English' or cereal. Porridge or toast? Pastries or bread and cheese and ham and preserves of all sorts. Marmalade was Daddy's favourite, the dark kind with thick chunks of rind in. I preferred 'silver shred' which was lighter and lemony and had tiny slivers of peel. Granda loved ginger marmalade and I could eat that by the spoonful. And I did. Later there were other breakfast discoveries. Croissants in France, Huevos Rancheros in Spain or New Mexico, peanut butter and jelly or pancakes. Dad wanted me to eat eggs at breakfast but I didn't like eggs.

Growing up, the dinner table didn't feel like a comfortable place to be. Often I didn't like the food. Boiled fish and onions. Boiled eggs. Tension. Manners. Saying the wrong thing. I announced that my period had started at the dining room table in front of my Mum, Dad and Granda. Mum had told me it was something to be proud of so I thought it was something to celebrate. There was a shocked silence and I knew I had got it wrong. I felt shamed and angry because I had been lied to again.

My place was to lay the table and make it nice. Sometimes I liked doing that when we had visitors. I liked to make the table look pretty and use the nice tablecloth and mats and glasses. It satisfied the artist in me. I still like to make the table pretty when it is an occasion. I like candles at Christmas and flowers at any time.

The table wasn't a relaxed place. Sometimes arguments started at the table. Tensions spilled out. Political differences. Religious conflicts. Misunderstandings. The table was a place of control and power. Who held the strings and who danced? Sometimes I fall into those old patterns. I see other people try to control the table and I start to mediate and distract. My stomach knots up and anxiety awakes from a half sleep. Sometimes it's easier to be alone.

At My Table

At my table
everyone is welcome
no-one is judged
we are all kind
everyone eats what they like
we can all talk
we laugh
we are relaxed
the food is good

Holding back my truth made me sick. I couldn't say how I felt because I didn't know unless you told me first. It made my voice small and then there would be a ball of fire that erupted like a volcano taking everyone with it. I got angry, depressed, fat and I kept feeling like there was something wrong with me. I couldn't live my whole real true life. It cost me my energy.

Being real means my body feels warm and safe. Sometimes it gets sick and my stomach hurts and I don't want to eat vegetables so I live on porridge and soup. Writing my first book made me sick as the trauma came up and out but it had to filter through the mesh of my life for me to see the damage and for the healing to begin.

My body is doing the work for my heart and my brain and it has so much to digest it needs easy food.

Meaning for me used to show up in cravings for sugar, alcohol and nicotine. When something was real and hard and big I wanted to hide away my feelings under a blanket of thick creamy sweetness. I wanted more of everything. The urge to consume told me I was feeling feelings that I couldn't feel. Consuming my feelings was safer than feeling them.

Today's meaning is warm in my body. Meaning is being able to take care of my needs.

Meaning is acknowledging these complex feelings deserve naming and feeling.

I took the words from our group and made this poem:

Cake

We want cake. We want to eat.

Carrot cake with cream cheese frosting

Birthday cake to keep us company

Sherry trifle surrounded by wobbly jelly, 'a complex dessert' she said, slightly tipsy

Sheet cake from the store, meant to cut and share

I want it all.

We want to eat cake.

Cake is for the sweetness and the longing

For the loneliness and the belonging

Cake to fill the hole we cannot fill

Cake to make it all better.

Cake to make us belong

It is the sweetness and the hit

It is checking out, numbing and blessed sleep

Butter yellow and only the best chocolate will do

Dark and rich and shiny, glossed over it sits on the tongue and slips down the throat

Not for me

The cheap kind is best, the sort that comes in purple family-sized packs

I am not worth the expensive stuff for my habit

Or maybe today I am

I need a treat

I need something just for me.

I hide my sugar treats in secret places

Stashes in drawers and cupboards and under the bed

The car is my safe place, my womb for eating it

Nurturing and sustaining me through the pain of living in this place I don't fit

I have my secrets

My supply to keep me safe

I am an addict

Sugar, food, alcohol, drugs, sex, shopping and more

They all fill a hole

But none ever did so much as food.

There is sticky spicy ginger cake with a cup of Earl Grey tea

Moist and fragrant and just for me

Binge sweet eaters

Freaks

Pigs

No we are not those words we call ourselves in shame and despair

We are adopted

I hate myself and yet I am finding

Here I am not alone

Its not just me

'Now I am sober' like a Christopher Robin story

No cake, drugs or booze

Sober is the new punk she said

I love that, I feel less of a freak

Diet Coke is too much of a drug for me now

And caffeine

I need to stay sober to be present

We help each other to be here

We are the survivors

We love each other

Cake for breakfast or in the wakeful hours of transatlantic time

Some of us are rich nutty fruit cake, redolent of Christmas spices and family celebrations

Heavy scents of cinnamon and cloves, thick white royal icing that my teeth sink into through that first crunch

Nuts may feature too and cheese and salty snacks in crinkly packets that rustle as we try

to eat them silently behind the door

Whipped or beaten cream, food is sensuous and seductive but I don't have time for the full

Experience

Just give me the hit forget the foreplay

Hoarding, shoveling, all in one go

Family interventions and sideways looks

We were tubby or skinny, food was love and love was food

Stealing, hoarding, keeping, seeking finding

It reminds us of what we long for most

Nature and nurture, both my mothers were addicted to sugar

A double whammy for me. Chocolate ran from her mouth like blood

Cake was our way to bond, ice cream and welsh cakes.

Pastries kept safe for 'emergencies' then eaten fast, they don't touch the sides

Cake as a care package

Cake as the placenta or are those handbags?

Feeding ourselves and each other

Nourished through Flourish

JULIA'S STORY:

I was brought up as an only child by my adoptive parents. I had some contact with the birth family including my mother until she died. I never made contact with my father and he has now passed on and I have been unable to find any relatives on that side. I was relinquished at six weeks old from a nursing home by my mother although she had limited contact with me and didn't want to see or hold me for the first few days as she had been told this would be easier (for her). My name at birth was Julia Anne. My name was changed to Fiona Margaret when I was adopted. I never felt right in my adopted name and I changed my first name back to Julia, keeping Fiona as a middle name as an act of keeping the peace. I was nearly 40 years old when I found my mother and biological siblings and I am now 63. My ongoing relationships with my biological family are complex. I wrote my story of adoption and recovery in Life In-Between (2021) and edited a compilation Dear Me with 12 women adoptees in 2022. I am no longer a child but I will always be an adoptee. I have complex feelings about adoption as an institution and also about my personal experience. For a very long time I had no idea that my feelings were what you might call 'normal' for someone who had been a) given away as a baby b) lived their life in a family that wasn't theirs. More and more people like me, i.e. adoptees, are clambering out of our respective closets and saying, "Here I am, this is my story, here is my voice.".

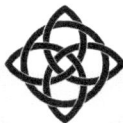

JULIA WINSTON
SOUTH CAROLINA

JOINING FLOURISH WAS THE FIRST TIME I had ever spent any substantive time, on purpose, with other adoptees. It was transformative for many reasons, one of them being the revelation that there were people who had something other than 'baby girl' or 'baby boy' on their original birth certificates — or OBC. I was born and adopted in South Carolina, where adoptee rights reform seems highly unlikely. I'd accepted the fact that the brief, censored non-ID information provided to my parents at my adoption would be the only official paperwork related to my origin that I would ever see. In Flourish, there were people from more progressive states who had their OBCs in hand. Several people in the group received their OBCs and learned their first names during the year, and that was a pretty powerful experience. Other people were in either past or present reunion with their bio fam and had learned their first names directly from them.

We were getting to know each other and feel out the group at the beginning of the year, but because of our connection through adoption we added questions like "public or private adoption?" and "What agency did your a-parents go through?" in addition to the usual questions of "Where do you live?" and "What do you do?"

As we continued talking the topic of original names came up, and I was surprised at how many group members knew that name. People got really excited and decided that everyone should change their names in the Flourish Zoom room to their original/birth names the next week. Looking back over my notes from the year, I found this scribbled at the top of the page for 2/24/21:

"I would rather strip naked and run into the chicken coop than keep staring at everyone's changed names on the Zoom chat."

(For a little bit of context, I was farm-sitting at the time and caring for four dogs, two cats, and 150 chickens. I'm terrified of birds and had a full head-to-

toe getup I donned to go into the chicken coop, even when I was there in the full heat of a Carolina summer.)

The next morning, I had my first tantrum in close to thirty years when recounting the experience to my therapist. I'm talking a full-on fist pounding, snot bubbling, "it's not fair" wailing tantrum. I don't think it was jealousy, exactly. I didn't want my new friends *not* to have that knowledge. I truly love my name, chosen carefully from family names on both sides of my family – I don't want another name. The whole experience was just another harsh reminder of something else that I had lost because of adoption.

I missed the next week because of school obligations (and probably at least a little avoidance) but made myself go back the next week, 3/10/21. We were talking about biosynthesis theory, and the ecto (skin, eyes, thinking), endo (organs, felt emotions), and meso (musculoskeletal system, movement) systems in the body. The writing prompt was: "Think about something related to the adoption experience – where are you in your systems?"

So, I wrote about names. *"Everything related to names and original names makes me feel so enraged I want to punch something or run away or cry, or maybe all three at the same time. I hate thinking about it. I hate seeing it. I hate seeing other people so happy and excited about it. And I then I feel like a shitty terrible person for feeling pain at other people's happiness and then I want to punch myself. It's the strongest physical reaction I've felt about anything in a long time.*

I don't know if I'm so angry because I know I don't have a so-called 'original name' and I'm jealous but rationally I don't want another name I love my name – my first name comes from my mom's favorite badass aunt and my middle name which is not only my father's name, it's my grandmother's name and I love the way it sounds and I don't want to change it.

Reading this out loud to the group may burn all of my bridges in the group and cut all ties and piss a bunch of people off, in which case it's been a cool few months and see y'all never! My jaw has been hurting all day and now crying about this has made my head hurt so now I'm fully miserable and want to _____ "

When it was my turn to share I seriously considered declining to read anything or at least ask to go later so that I could craft something else without the possibility of hurting other group members (It's such an adoptee thing to put everyone else's potential hurt feelings ahead of my own actual feelings). But something inside me said that maybe it might not go as poorly as what I'd played out in my head, so I blew my nose and went for it. I started with my final 'see y'all never' disclaimer, followed by the next two paragraphs. Then, I waited. Held my breath and waited for the metaphorical pitchforks.

The pitchforks never came. The private chat messages did – messages of comfort and commiseration. I felt valued and supported because I had shared, not in spite of it. This pattern continued throughout several more of my meltdowns over the year. I would get vulnerable and say something expecting to be reviled, only to be embraced instead. The tiny strangers on the Wednesday night Zoom meetings became people, and then friends, and then family members as we shared our way through things as silly as a board game proposal to as serious as the nothing place.

JULIA'S STORY:

I was relinquished at birth in South Carolina. I spent my first three days in a hospital, my first three weeks with a foster family, then was placed with my third mother (and father), my adoptive parents. I was raised as an only child. I don't have my original birth certificate and am not currently in reunion.

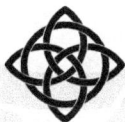

KARRI

WASHINGTON

Questions for my First Mother

I FOUND MY FIRST MOTHER when I was 36. I had a lot of mystery around her from an early age. I was not given a lot of information growing up. My parents had the standard adoption paperwork and I was never allowed to look at it.

I have a handful of letters that my first mother wrote me in the two years we were in contact. She would write and I would write back the next day. I would check the mail obsessively. I would wait weeks for another letter to come. Her letters were sporadic at best. In two years I received five letters. When the letters did come I would save them until I had some quiet time to take it all in, to savor every word from her.

I wanted more. I tried not to beg, but I was hungry for information and I longed to know her. If I knew the right questions to ask she would answer them. At the time I didn't know what my future self would want answers to and I had no idea our time would be cut so short.

I found out she had passed away by a message left by her daughter with my young son while I was at an appointment. Her daughter had found my letters I wrote and called. I couldn't believe it. She was gone, just like that. I have grieved this woman I never knew. She was 59, too young to die. I wish I had known that her death was so close, closer than even she knew I think. What I want now are more details surrounding my birth day. I want what most people take for granted.

One week in Flourish the prompt was to write questions for our first mother. I wrote my questions to someone I had only seen in pictures and I spoke to her as I read to the group. I could barely get through the questions without choking up, forgetting that 25 people were watching me as I read.

I won't ever get answers but I can tell you to ask the questions when you can, you never know how long you have.

These were some of my questions from that night:

What was your relationship like with my biological father?

What did you do after you found out you were pregnant?

Who helped you during your pregnancy?

Did you work? Where?

Were you harassed for being single and pregnant?

What were your favorite foods while pregnant?

What was your pregnancy like? Did you talk or sing to me?

What was the day of my birth like for you and me?

What time of day was I born?

What did you feel like when you got the call from the intermediary I hired to find you?

Why didn't you tell your family about me? At the time or when you knew I had located you?

Did you know dying was a possibility when we were writing letters?

Do you have regrets?

Do you know that I would have done anything to see you?

I miss you.

Flourish

Being adopted has been a complex mix of emotions and behaviors for most of my life. I feel like I have been trying to figure out relationships ever since birth when my most important one was severed. My relationships, no matter how superficial or serious have always felt awkward and disconnected. I thought I was broken. I thought I was the only one that felt this way. I felt so alone much of the time.

Adoption has ruined a lot of things for me, how I attach to people, trust, safety, communication, relationships, self-esteem, confidence and love. Often I looked for connection in all the wrong places for all the wrong reasons.

Talking to non adoptees about my experiences was difficult because I didn't feel as if I was free to be my full, true self. I left a lot of my story out to make sure others were comfortable. Not sharing becomes normal and the easiest way to survive but there was an expense to my mind and body. There are so many secrets and lies that come with adoption. Once my mom asked me "Why do you have to tell everyone you're adopted?" I knew after that to not talk about being adopted to anyone outside of our house, it was a shameful secret. This led to me having to keep up with my mom's stories about who I looked like most, her or my dad? Not being able to tell the truth when someone would comment on a similar personality trait I seemed to share. I wanted to be able to tell the story that I was "special" or "chosen" like they said I was. Integrity and truth are my favorite traits now.

In the spring of 2018 I found the *Adoptees On* podcast and this opened the door to a world of adopted people I had no idea existed. I heard people on the podcast telling a similar story to mine. Hearing people just like me was what I needed. I knew I wanted to meet these people.

I heard about a retreat hosted by Anne and Pam in the fall 2018. I had to find a way to go. Oh, to be in a room with other adoptees. These were my people, I could relate in some way to everyone there. I was hooked on finding more of the adoptee community. The safety and trust I felt at the retreat was like a drug I had never had. My soul needed that. I remember saying that I could live in that safe place forever. I still have close friends from that retreat, we actually call ourselves sisters because that's what the relationship feels like to us. When we talk, we share as if we are teenagers, laughing and confiding about things others don't understand, a relationship I haven't had with any one of my seven siblings.

Fast forward to fall 2020: I heard about a Flourish class, it sounded interesting, it was a drop-in group at that time. I believed whole heartedly in what the intention of the group was. Pam and Anne wanted to create friendships like they had together. They wanted to create more community! I was IN! On my own Instagram I promoted it and even offered to pay for a few people to try it out. I wanted other adoptees to have friends like I had found and I wanted to meet more people. We need other adopted people in our lives. We need safe places where we can trust each other. We need a place to have our humor and spill our tears over the rejection we feel.

In January, it became a yearlong commitment, same people (and their dogs, some cats) every week. There were a few people I already knew but most were new faces to me. At first it was uncomfortable for me to talk in front of so many people. I get nervous, I sweat, and I don't think I sound like I know what I am talking about in large groups. A year was a long time to commit to, but I knew

I wanted to be on the ground floor of this Flourish whatever it was going to be. I trusted Anne and Pam to keep it a safe place for me and they did. I was not disappointed.

I found in Flourish that every week, I had a receptive place to go. I could be seen, heard and understood without any explanation. A lot between us was unspoken, we knew we shared the same mother loss and that was all there was, that was all there needed to be.

It was hard emotional work some weeks and in the end I learned so much about myself.

For instance, I wasn't comfortable with my answers to some of the prompts and would find myself second guessing, I couldn't relax until I heard others speak their answers. I wanted to know mine was just as good. Learning to trust my instincts, go with my gut was a big bonus from Flourish. I am just as good as the others. I gained confidence and this has spilled over in other parts of my life with work and my relationships. I speak up a lot more and say what I feel, I trust my own judgment more.

I also learned when I want to be funny is usually at a time when I am feeling uncomfortable with something that is digging deep inside that I don't want to touch. It was a coping mechanism and my way to fit in. I started looking at those times and what it was that made me want to joke myself out of the conversation or throw off the attention to laughter. I learned that I can be funny, it can be appreciated and I could safely be vulnerable in Flourish without it. This group of people showed me they could hold me in an emotional situation.

I talked about my relationship with my son, the awkwardness I have with my adoptive parents, the estrangement from my adoptive brother and working through matters regarding my biological family. All of it I brought to Wednesday nights. No holding back, most of what I shared in Flourish I had never shared before. I found hope and understanding from everyone, there was empathy because we all knew what this was like for each other. It was incredible to see the head shakes in agreement as others spoke. I found a belonging.

There were fun times where we would all just bust up laughing so hard there were tears, there were sad times and there were bumpy, hard times. I learned that you can stay and work it out. I had always cut and run, the first to leave when the going got tough or things were upsetting, I was glad for the example of staying with it and working the problem out.

I will always be adopted, but I have the courage and community to forge ahead with my new tools and knowledge of self.

As Pam says "We heal in community."

I encourage you to find yours as I have.

KARRI'S STORY:

I was adopted 18 days after birth through the Children's Home Society of Washington. I was raised with a non-related adopted brother, two years younger than me. I have six other siblings, three from my first mother and three from my biological father, one sister is three months younger than me. I am in contact with one of my siblings at this time, my adopted sister. I began the process of finding my biological family at 36 years old. My first mother passed away two years after contact in 2001 and I never met her. Bio father and I maintain a cordial relationship. My earliest memory of being told I was adopted is age 11. I was not named by my mother but was given the name Linda in foster care while I waited for adoption. My parents named me Karri.

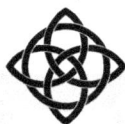

KATIE KENNEDY

MINNESOTA

What has Flourish Meant to Me?

I WAS SCROLLING ON MY PHONE in early December 2020, as I frequently did during the pandemic, when I saw a blog post from Anne Heffron about a weekly class she and her friend Pam Cordano were facilitating in the new year. I have followed Anne's blog since finding my birth family and reading her book, *You Don't Look Adopted*, as she was the first person who put words to feelings I've carried my entire life. In this particular blog post, she wrote of her thoughts about Flourish, a yearlong commitment for 20 adoptees to learn and grow together in community. Anne wrote, "Both are about community and love. And you." Hmmmm, community, love and me, what could possibly go wrong? I had never done anything like this, yet I knew I had to do it. My whole body was saying yes in spite of all the unknowns. The normal rush of anxiety telling me to back away, don't do it, this is not safe, was strangely missing. Instead, I was excited. I was eager and I wanted to learn from, and be with, other adoptees. I couldn't wait to sign up. I emailed Anne that night and joined Flourish. It was likely the best email I have ever sent.

A little backstory on me: I wasn't born, I arrived. I arrived three-and-a-half weeks after my alleged birth without any information about the supposed woman who gave birth to me or her family, or a man. Nothing about her pregnancy, where my birth took place or even if a doctor was present. No vital statistics. Nothing.

To make things more confusing, there was a document titled "Certificate of Live Birth" which claims I was born to my parents. Very strange indeed since my parents were not able to conceive children. Yet, it is a legal document that is certified by the Minnesota State Board of Health, so it must be true, right? It unequivocally states that I am theirs, yet I'm still fairly certain there wasn't an actual 'live' birth. Surely if there were I would have heard a story or two about it, and there were no stories of birthing going on in my family. What I did have was a story about the day I arrived. What a glorious day it was, my parents and brothers welcomed me, and now our family was complete.

I recall talk of a woman who loved me so much she wanted to give me to my parents. Finally I had a story to tell my fellow classmates who were always asking about my real parents. I felt so bad for those poor kids that were kept, their parents didn't get to choose them. My parents DID choose me, AND that woman loved me so much she let them have me. Now that is a good story, and it's all mine. Well, actually, my brothers have the same story and who are we to argue with any of it, after all, we are so lucky to have arrived at our parents.

Come to find out I actually was born. My birthday was a day to be celebrated, yet my birth remained a mystery. There WAS this other woman (and a man, neither of which are ever to be discussed) and she did give me to my parents, via the Catholic Church. This event, like my birth and all events leading to my birth, are to be hidden as they are very, very shameful and riddled with sin. I wonder what parts of me are full of sin and what parts of me should be hidden in shame. Instinctively, I knew I should never find these alleged parents as it would only cause more shame and immeasurable hurt. I should, and do, count my lucky stars I am not being raised by 'those' people.

This arrival thing called adoption can be pretty confusing and heartbreaking to a young person. Quite frankly, I am still pretty confused and heartbroken about it decades later.

And now, I find myself in my first Flourish class with Anne Heffron talking about being a continuous person. Interesting concept, especially since I don't feel continuous. How can I be with a history so full of stories, secrets, shame and nothingness?

Anne talked about how our hands can be our cohesive narrative when we don't feel connected. She asked us to look at our hands. To spend time really looking at our hands, and then write about what it feels like to look at them knowing they were inside of our mother. Whoa. Now that may seem like a crazy thought to normal people (another thing I learned in Flourish is we all call people who were kept, normal). But, when you've had your heritage, identity, family and first chapter erased, it becomes a very reasonable and interesting thought. I get it. I completely understand not feeling whole or connected.

My life had a significant break when I was relinquished by my mother. I can't imagine a bigger trauma for an infant or young child. I will never know my birth story, and I will never know my mother. I have lived with an underlying feeling of not being real, authentic or quite right. How could I be whole and continuous when I didn't have anything except a big black hole of nothingness to tell me who I was?

I didn't see proof of my birth until I was 58 years old when I received my *original* "Certificate of Live Birth" and it was a lot different from my *legal* "Certificate of Live Birth."

Finally the truth. I really was born in a hospital, with a doctor, at 5:58 a.m. I was weighed and measured and my mother had a real name and address. I still didn't have a father, but I had a name! She gave me a name, so that must mean she loved me, right? Oh, and there was a new box that was checked called, "illegitimate." What a cruel and heartless thing to label an innocent child. I am purposefully not swearing here so I deleted my initial reaction to that word. You can use your imagination or stick with cruel and heartless, either way, nothing can accurately describe the awfulness of that word.

I was a part of my mother, hands and all. Her body nourished and loved me, my hands and body grew and moved inside her, I knew her heartbeat and the energy of her. She had me baptized, and the Church falsified those records in an attempt to erase and minimize her, and our bond.

Parents are sacred, they are not to be erased. She was real, and nothing can remove her from my life and my being, not even her death. Our time together was short, yet there is so much shared history with a woman I wasn't permitted to know.

Her name was Grace, and I am her daughter.

I feel mostly sadness when reflecting on Anne's question, along with comfort that, even with everything I lost, I am a continuous being and I am whole.

Yet I still wonder...

> *I wonder if my hands reached for my mother when she held me for the first and last time.*
>
> *I wonder if my little fingers wrapped themselves around her fingers before she left.*
>
> *I wonder if my hands touched her face.*
>
> *I wonder if she kissed my hands.*
>
> *I wonder if my hands instinctively moved toward her breasts in search of nourishment.*

I didn't know she was leaving. I imagine I felt so safe and secure in those sacred moments while she held me. When I was hers and she was mine.

I wonder what part of me died the day she left.

Grace's baby ceased to exist the day Grace walked out of that hospital, and the remaining part of me arrived at my parents three-and-a-half weeks later. My little hands kept searching for my mother while she was being erased from my life. Why would I ever want to delve into such a deep and painful separation? I avoided it for decades, until finding my first family, and Anne's question that first night in Flourish. Thinking of, and speaking about, being born to and being physically inside of someone you have never met is quite overwhelming and very painful...and also very healing.

My answer was short and simple:

I wish my hands could talk and tell me about my beginnings.

I wish they could fill in the missing pieces and tell me about my mother and why

she left me.

I wish they could tell me what being loved by my mother feels like.

This was my beginning with Flourish and the start of the most healing year of my life.

The writing prompts were sensitive and thought provoking and led me to a place of personal understanding and growth. It is difficult to answer these questions and more difficult to read them out loud to a zoom screen filled with strangers. Week after week we read to each other. I cried when I read my answer to that first question, and was more touched when my fellow flourishers read their responses. Some were funny, some were sad, some were angry and they all had the same undertone of longing and grief. This became a pattern, week after week, we all shared eerily similar feelings and responses.

For the first time in my life, I didn't feel like I was different, instead my deepest feelings were validated. Flourish made me feel real. I wasn't alone. After all, they too have lived with the stories of their arrivals and not their births. They too, have lost everything.

Later in that first class, Anne asked if we could write a prayer on our skin, what would it say?

I wrote:

I am enough

I am worthy

Be still

Trust

I get very emotional thinking about that night and every Wednesday night since. One year later, I would write the same prayer on my skin, and add a prayer to include other adoptees who, like myself, have buried their grief and emotions. I pray that all relinquished and adopted people find a community of other adoptees to feel the sense of calm, understanding, love and trust that I have found with Flourish. I now have a community of people who understand, who nod their heads when I speak of things others can't fathom. It feels like home and family, and that is something to celebrate.

KATIE'S STORY:

I was relinquished at birth to Catholic Charities and stayed with them until going to my parents at three-and-a-half weeks old. I was raised with two, nonbiological, older brothers who were also adopted through Catholic Charities. I always knew I was adopted; my brothers and I imagined that we all had the same mother. We were also told that our parents would support us if we decided to search for our biological families, yet most of my questions were met with tears, so I stopped asking. I confidentially requested my non-identifying information when I was in my early 20's. I grew up dreaming that my biological parents were looking for me, which I found to be both terrifying and exhilarating, and was devastated to find this was not the case.

My biological mother named me Sheri Ann and I was baptized five days after my birth. Along with my birth certificate, my baptismal certificate was legally falsified to reflect my new existence, my new name and my new parents.

I found my biological mother and father when I was 55 years old by doing Ancestry and 23andMe. Unfortunately, my biological mom had passed away the previous year. I am told that she wrote the following poem about me one night after a walk. I cherish these words as they are all I have to know that she thought about me and loved me.

"Last night I had a dream of peace,

as I walked in darkness

the stars shined upon me

I wondered which one was put there for you

and as I looked

there it was

smiling bright at me."

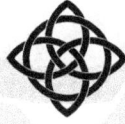

KIRSTEN WEATHERFORD
MONTANA

FLOURISH: *The safest space to pour out all your shit and know that everyone else understands the stench.*

I wrote that early in our time together. It was before the one-year commitment had even started, but the magic of what could happen was evident. There is healing in community. When adoptees feel seen and heard – truly valued – it is powerful. For the first time in my life, I let down my guard. Week after week, I would show up, knowing full well that it may be a difficult two hours to get through. I kept showing up because even when it was hard, when my emotions were overflowing and I felt raked over the coals, I never felt alone. People would reach out and check in on me. There were personal messages of understanding and encouragement. In the times it was the hardest, that was where I grew the most. In looking back, it truly is amazing to see what we accomplished in our time together. Through the laughter, tears, truth, and vulnerability shared in Flourish, I am a changed person.

When I went back through my notes, I found different snippets that struck me. Sometimes, they were full writings. Other times, they were simple sentences. No matter the length of the passage, the power was tangible. "Aha!" moments happened all the time, often when least expected. That was the power of being in community. Sometimes all it took was a person to say the "right" thing, and the faces on the screen would change. People would nod in agreement, and collective tears might flow. Sometimes, it was just hearing my own voice speaking my truth that brought the gut punch and the raw emotion. But every single time it happened, I would grow a little bit. I would shed another layer of my cocoon in anticipation of someday flying free.

January's theme was "belonging," and I saw a lot of emotion there in looking back over my notes. January is also my birthday month, and birthdays are complicated for adoptees. One night in particular, all three of the writing prompts seemed to be exactly what I needed.

What was the first time you remember feeling like you didn't belong?

"I was riding in the back seat of our car, traveling to visit my grandparents. I was missing a few days of school while we traveled, so I had homework that had been sent with me. I was supposed to draw a picture each day to document what was happening. Every time I looked down to try and draw in the car, I felt like I was going to puke. My mother accused me of lying and simply not wanting to do the work. She told me I was lazy and was making excuses because I wanted to sleep in the car instead of doing my homework. I was five years old."

In the minutes I spent responding to the prompt, I became that five-year-old little girl again, nausea included. Except now I felt sick because of the way I'd been spoken to, not because of having motion sickness. I was processing what had been said from my adult perspective, and I visualized holding my five-year-old self and telling her I believed her. She really did feel sick trying to read or write in the car. That's something that continued throughout her life. Just because her adoptive mom could read entire novels on car trips and she couldn't didn't mean something was wrong with her. And the trips that she did end up puking in the car? Those could be considered little gifts for the mother who thought she was making it all up.

What was the "fatal flaw" you told yourself of why you were relinquished?

"I was repeatedly told that I was the product of my young birth mom's affair with a married man. She was trashy – and since I was the product of that affair – I was trash, too. That's why I was thrown away like unwanted garbage."

I spent my childhood hearing the story of my conception repeated over and over. It seemed to be one of the ways my adoptive parents could show their one-up-manship. It served as proof of their superiority, not only as people in a committed relationship, but also their deemed worthiness as parents. It fed their narrative, and that of society, that they had saved me and given me a better life. I was given a different life, but not necessarily a better one. Writing those words out on paper made me physically examine them. Once I wrote them out and dissected them, they lost their power. That was my adoptive parents version of the story, but I was learning to no longer make it mine. The facts were there; I was the product of an affair. That act had nothing to do with my right to take up space in the world. And I was not doomed to an existence as sub-human.

Where do you yearn to belong?

"I yearn to belong in my own body. I want to not hate the person who stares back at me from the mirror. I don't know her, and I don't really like anything about her. She is a stranger in spite of the fifty years we have shared together."

Body image has been a struggle my entire life. In my teen years, I was really good at not feeding myself. As an adult, it's the opposite problem. Either way, it's about struggling to love my own image and seeing the truth of the reflection in the mirror. Prior to reunion with my biological mom, I had no idea what my family looked like. I now know that some of my battles are pointless. I've been attempting to fight my own DNA. I'm still trying to learn how to love the body I live in.

The theme for February was mutuality. The last week of the month was about risk and reward.

What risks aren't I taking?

"I shrink back from anything that feels like drawing attention to myself. I try to stay small – unseen and unheard, otherwise it feels like having to admit I have a right to take up space and exist. I avoid anything that feels like self-promotion. I prefer to stay small and unnoticed – which most people who know me (outside of my family) would have a hard time believing. I project a confident, secure persona while I am internally hustling to try and get it all right."

After I read my response to the prompt to the group, Anne pushed me to dig a little deeper. She asked me to read my response again, and asked what was uncomfortable about having to admit I have a right to exist. It was an epiphany, albeit a painful one. By admitting I have a right to be alive, I also had to admit that I don't always feel that way, and that I still want to die sometimes. Those feelings, in spite of hard work to heal and unravel everything that adoption has programmed me to believe, are still lurking just below the surface. And some days, I don't have to go very far to reach them. But the growth I gained in Flourish helps me identify what is really happening in those dark moments. I've slipped into "The Nothing Place." It's the darkness only adoptees truly know. I now know there are others I can reach out to from that darkness who understand beyond words, and who will sit with me until I can see the light again.

It was an honor to be part of such a groundbreaking concept. Anne and Pam understood the profound power of their own friendship. From that friendship, the idea of "Flourish" was born. From my understanding, their vision was to see other adoptees thrive and heal together in a supportive setting. We would all understand each other from the outset, because of our shared experiences and common ground as adoptees. There were many weeks that the work we did was hard. Exhausting, even. But working through the hard stuff in a group setting, where so many could identify with the exact feelings one of us was working through, made it doable. I never felt alone, and I felt seen and understood in ways that I'd never experienced before. Finding mutual understanding among other adoptees provided opportunities for growth that would have been exponentially more difficult to navigate on my own. I am grateful for the growth I experienced due to Flourish, and for the beautiful women whose vision spawned the idea.

KIRSTEN'S STORY:

I was born in Pennsylvania toward the tail-end of the Baby Scoop Era early in 1971. I was relinquished to the county/state immediately at birth. With the day's prevailing belief being that mother-infant bonding occurred after birth, my first mother never saw me or held me. She was told it was "best" for both of us. I spent a week in the hospital, and nearly three months in foster care before being placed with my adoptive parents. I was raised as an only child. In spite of their best efforts to shape and mold the "blank slate" baby they'd been given, we were never the right fit for each other. At the age of 39, I began to understand what impact adoption has had on my life. Nothing has been the same since. When I was 46, I found the maternal side of my first family. We have been in reunion for five years. Soon after that reunion, the relationship with my adoptive parents completely broke. It had been decades in the making. My refusal to remain the good, loyal, indebted adoptee was too much for them, and I was dismissed.

In recent years, I've found enduring friendships in the adoptee community. The voices I first discovered through the Adoptees On podcast brought me comfort, validation, and grounding. Flourish helped tether my wandering soul and cemented a belief that what I have to say holds value. Thus far, I've been a guest on two adoptee podcasts, started a blog, and published a book. I've just begun to tell my story, and there is more yet to come.

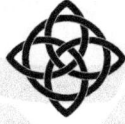

LORA K. JOY

INDIANA

Flourishing

FOR TWELVE YEARS after realizing my adoption trauma, I thought I was the only person in the world to feel this pain and loneliness. Fortunately, in 2020, through the *Adoptees On* podcast, I found this amazing community. I reached out to Anne Heffron to be my writing coach and jumped in, continuing to make connections. When Anne told me about her and Pam's idea for Flourish, I signed up immediately. The first couple of classes were about addiction, something that I did not struggle with, but I decided to show up anyway. It is so amazing that even though addiction was not my lived experience, I learned so much from that first class.

Pam and Anne wanted to see what would happen if a group of adoptees spent a year together, writing, sharing and healing. For me, the answer at the end of that year was I had a family. My Flourish family is truly the first place I have ever belonged and felt I could show up raw, honest and complete in my authenticity. This group has become my church. We all feel seen and understood without needing to explain our emotions. There is magic in connecting so deeply with a group of adoptees. We are mirrors for each other like no one else can be. Together we uncover our truth – that and the rawness, deep honesty and reflection is where you find the power and healing.

This book project is meant to encourage others to find their "Flourish Family." We want other adoptees to heal and find community the way we have. It is hard to put language to our experience. I walked this earth for 41 years before I found my fellow Flourishers and I honestly don't know how I survived. In the people in Flourish, I have found unconditional love, attunement, the feeling of being cared for, mirrors, understanding without explanation and a place I belong. I walk differently in the world now because I carry my fellow Flourishers with me.

Aside from the weekly writing prompts, Flourish has provided myself and many others a safe place to explore reclaiming our lives. One example is that I legally changed my name to my birth name, Lora. Flourish was the first place I "tried on" my birth name. I started showing up in this space as Lora. Everyone understood without explanation the complexity of multiple names, of denouncing the name that never felt right – the name that felt like a lie every time you said it or answered to it. As time went on I started to realize I was no longer my adoptive name, I was Lora – who I always should have been. If I did not have Flourish, I'm not sure I ever would have been brave enough or had the space to shed this layer of adoption trauma.

Through all my internal work on adoption, I have come to realize that I existed in a dysregulated state until I found Flourish. The healing from this group regulated my system – allowing me for the first time to interact with others and the world in a more appropriate way.

Flourish was not therapy, but a lot of my healing has happened in this place. The first weekly prompt that broke me open was Womb Writings. We were to write a message to our birth mothers from inside the womb. Think of it like graffiti or leaving our mark on our first home, likely for a lot of us, the last place we ever felt safe.

Writing my own messages was unbelievably difficult and painful. It was everything I wish I could have changed about the circumstances that led to my adoption. As other members of the group shared, I cried, and I barely choked through what I had written.

I love you.

I'm excited to meet you.

Why are you so sad?

I can't wait to meet my brother and help you take care of him.

My dad lied to you. He's 47 and his other children are 17 and 12.

Don't listen to your mother. I need to stay with you. Please don't give me to strangers.

I'm sorry my dad left you, but we will be OK as long as we are together.

As everyone continued to read aloud, one member spoke up, "if the world could hear all of us, adoption would be abolished."

We were all babies speaking from the womb, but with the hindsight of knowing what a lifetime of being adopted meant. We were leaving our mark to say we existed.

If the world could see our pain, would they change the happy narrative of adoption? Would it give future birth mothers pause to know their babies need and want only them?

I sometimes think about the womb being my wound, but it really was my first and last safe place.

⊗

Adoptive Babies Cries

IF MY WOMB WRITING communicates that I was so desperate to stay with my mother, what did I say when I was taken away from her? What did I say to a foster mother, then my adoptive mother?

My body tensed and I was scared. I felt and knew I was not safe or where I belonged. The person who took care of me at the "tender care" home and my adoptive mother were the wrong people to hold me and give me what I needed.

Fellow adoptee Lauren Zoller wrote a powerful blog piece that included responses to her adoptive mother. Her words felt like they were taken from the ends of my cries, like she had read my heart when I was a baby:

"Who are you?

I'm not yours.

You are not mine.

Don't touch me.

I want to leave.

I don't belong here."

I would add *"I don't understand you."*

Babies need their biological mothers. An adoptive mother is not a sufficient replacement.

Secure in The Nothing Place

THE NOTHING PLACE.

Where I arrived when I lost my mother moments after birth.

Where I have lived and the place I know well.

The place I reject the woman who tries to take her place.

No one understands this place. I am all alone.

Floating in a void.

Untethered.

There is a black hole between me and the rest of the world.

Home.

Relax, You're Home

I have been alone my whole life – from the moment I was taken from my mother at birth. It did not matter that a foster parent took care of me for five weeks. It did not matter that I was placed with adoptive parents. No one could replace my biological mother.

Losing her catapulted me out into a void where I have lived and operated from ever since.

Walking through life, I knew I was different. I was in the wrong place; I was with strangers. No one understood me. Everyone around me had a mother, knew what it was like to be given unconditional love, to be understood, to be mirrored, to know their place.

I was always looking across this void, longingly, wishing I could be a part of that world.

When I had my children, I gave them everything I wished I had. Which only brought into sharper focus what I was missing – what I could never have.

Pam discovered this place on her own journey and named it – The Nothing Place. She brought that revelation to Flourish and named it for the rest of us. Once she explained what The Nothing Place was, there was a collective relaxation in our group. Everyone understood and we were all there together.

It seems no one can understand The Nothing Place except other adoptees. We recognize the black hole, the deafening silence. The Nothing Place is my home, my beginning and while I have lived my whole life here alone, I am now finding community and strength with other adoptees that call this place home too.

Flourish gave me community and context for my lived experience. It gave me the opportunity to be with other people who understood me. As an adoptee I had never had this immediate sense of belonging before. Being with other adoptees only pointed out more of what I had been missing my entire life and once I had that understanding, I did not want to waste my energy with other people who didn't understand or with people I couldn't be my authentic self.

I have decided I would rather be alone than with others who do not understand or who only want to view my experience from their own perspective and expectations. In The Nothing Place, I have built strength, community and resilience to survive. Adoptees deserve to have agency in their lives and Flourish gave me the strength and fortitude to reclaim my life.

Now that I know the name of the place I live and understand how I got there, I am embracing it. The Nothing Place is home because that is where I am, the only person I have ever been able to depend on.

THE NOTHING PLACE = HOME.
Fellow adoptees are always welcome.

LORA'S STORY:

I was relinquished at birth and adopted at five weeks old through a Catholic agency. I was raised as an only child and learned I was adopted when I was eight years old. My adoptive name was Joy, but I have reclaimed my birth name of Lora. I am fully estranged from my adoptive family and experienced secondary rejection from my biological father. I am in successful reunion with my biological mom and brother as well as paternal siblings and cousins.

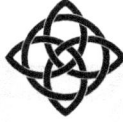

MICHELLE MADSEN HINTON

Belonging

I AM 46 AND STILL AFRAID to speak my whole truth. I can honestly say I have never really had a sense of belonging. I was in attendance. I was around others, yet found I felt lost and alone. That feeling convinced me I wasn't worthy of belonging.

Coming out of the fog of the societal expectations of adoption can be liberating and soul crushing. Adoption is beautiful, to most unadopted people. However, as an adoptee, the trauma, loneliness, sadness will catch you and steal your breath. The effect of adoption on my life is all encompassing. It wasn't a single event. It wasn't a single court date, or "gotcha day." I live it daily and can reflect on how it showed up in the past. Truth is, I was not the first choice. I was no one's first choice. I don't belong.

To sit down and write about my experience as an adoptee is hard. It's hard to explain and hard to hear. I know people may take offense. They are the ones who need to listen the most. It's not about you. I've written and erased pages of disjointed paragraphs, concerned I wasn't making sense. Which is exactly right. Living as an adoptee is so disordered.

How do I convey the duality of adoption to others? The holding of two seemingly opposite truths at the same time can feel impossible, even annihilating. Recently I have begun an attempt to educate and convey the trauma of adoption and lived abandonment. Most don't want to really listen or learn. Exploring the effects of trauma on infants –and lifelong trauma – requires learning and educating parents, family, loved ones, and practitioners. But that requires communication. And it has rarely happened.

Truth: I love my family. Period. Full stop.

Truth: I hate the trauma of relinquishment that created it.

Reality: I had to lose everything to be in my family.

This loss is stored in our brains and bodies and shows up later in a myriad of ways.

I have felt this abandonment my whole life. I have stayed in relationships and friendships that were abusive, in order to feel kept.

Brain: *I will be left again. If I am not good enough, they will leave. If I don't behave, they will leave. I was left before, why wouldn't it happen again?* This taught me that love equals leaving.

One of my first memories is an example of the effect. When I was four years old, I was so excited to start preschool. The in-home preschool was a few blocks from home. We practiced walking there and back. The big day came for me to walk to school by myself, and by the time I got a third of the way there I was terrified and sobbing uncontrollably. I could no longer see my house; I would never see my parents again. I was positive. They left. I ran home sobbing, and my mom couldn't figure out what was wrong... how was I to communicate that terror I felt at four years old? Even adults don't have the words, and most won't talk about it. Thus began an extensive list of events where I had no way to explain what was wrong. So, in essence, I was wrong. My parents thought I was shy, needed to be pushed, overreacting and too sensitive. I tried to be more than I was, be more outgoing, and more self-confident. Unfortunately, you just can't wish yourself out of trauma. There are a few people in my life that try so hard to understand, my husband most of all. But it is not possible to understand, they can only imagine. But empathy is not a trait everyone can show.

I can't tell you how many mental health "disorders" I have been labeled with, or how many prescriptions I have tried to "fix" myself. So many pills. So many doctors. Problem is, it's all a misplaced Band-Aid, and I feel like a gaping wound. Why didn't others see it? How do I just "get over it"?

I am not broken. I have no "fatal flaw" that makes me unlovable. However, my brain has convinced me I am wrong, bad, unworthy. A parent would only leave if I was bad, right? And unfortunately, society has perpetuated this false narrative. If I am not grateful, I am the problem. How many other devastating life traumas are people expected to be thankful for? Yet, when I speak of how it has affected me, I am shut down, told I am just an angry, ungrateful adoptee. An ungrateful little brat.

As a 40-something adult, I felt unmoored. My neurological system was on fire, and I had to find out why. In 2020 I took a deep dive into the adoptee world. I needed to know I wasn't alone, the only one who felt like this. I listened to podcasts, read every book and journal article I could find. Honestly, I was frantic. Nothing I had been doing to treat my anxiety, depression, agoraphobia, was working. I had to know what was wrong with me! I have learned there was never anything wrong with me ... my reaction was normal for the abnormal situation.

All those labels before were just symptoms of Complex-PTSD. All my worst fears happened before I had a voice. I was abandoned.

The pandemic created an opportunity for accessibility to online communities. I discovered a weekly Zoom meet-up for adoptees. It was fucking magical! Over the past 17 months, I have been surrounded by this amazing group of adoptees, who are more like family, sacred friends. We discuss and write on topics related to relinquishment and adoptee trauma. We talk about the hard stuff. I have come to know what true belonging feels like. I am seen as I am, without question, heard without debate, never told to shut up, and never ever ignored. Each member of Flourish grants me grace, healing, understanding, and a place where I am safe to fall apart. We are a network of people that fiercely protect each other. Our pain is acknowledged and can be grieved in community. The beautiful faces I see weekly reflect with understanding. In essence we mirror each other's truth. Mirroring our collective experiences, all so varied but with one constant, we had all been relinquished. We all know that pain and grief. Together we can heal. My internal alarm system has been blaring for 46 years. They helped me lower the volume.

It is an enormous gift, belonging.

MICHELLE'S STORY:

I was born to a 17-year-old, eight weeks premature, and relinquished to social services. My adoption court documents state I was born out of wedlock, illegitimate, and my only name was "baby girl." I've never seen my original birth certificate. After birth I remained in an incubator, in the NICU for two months. No kangaroo care, no biological recall, smell, feel; alone. I still can't acknowledge that the baby was me. I was released to my adoptive parents' care from the hospital. Less than a year later my adoptive parents welcomed their biological daughter, my little sister. I have always known I was adopted. I was told that it didn't matter, and we sure didn't talk about it.

At age 19 I was surprised into reunion with my biological father and most of my paternal family. My biological parents married after I was born, and had two more daughters, eight and ten years younger than me. My biological mother passed away when I was 11, we never met. Nine years later my older sister found our biological father. Two adoptees in one family. I am in contact with some biological family, some have since rejected me. This is what makes being an adoptee so fucking hard. I must protect everyone's feelings while ignoring my own. I have been juggling everyone's feelings for so long that when I started to express my truth, I angered a lot of people.

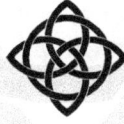

MONIQUE FLORENCE SARAH PANGARI

AUSTRALIA

Fantasy vs Reality

I FOUND OUT THAT I HAD BEEN ADOPTED while sitting in the back seat of my parents Ford Falcon when I was about five years old. We were off on our annual family vacation to the Gold Coast. I was squished in the middle, with a brother on either side of me. I hated those road trips. I usually had a window seat because my eldest brother and I fought too much to be able to sit next to one another and my parents had to separate us.

We were all adopted. Max was the eldest, four years older than me and Anthony was in the middle, two years older than me. I was the youngest and the only girl. Max and I had never gotten along. We had nothing in common.

I remember the big announcement. We were driving through Nambour and Dad declared, "This is where we got you from, Monique." Those words 'got you from' still echo in my mind today. He went on to explain that all three of us were 'adopted.' He didn't explain much more than that, there were some words about your mother not being your mother. Mum stared ahead at the road, we sat quietly in the back. No real explanation, no eye contact, no soothing words, no questions, no answers. I knew something was not good about this. Everything felt different after that. I guess what I came to understand was that I was born in that town to a different mother and my brothers also had another set of parents too, ones we knew nothing about, ones we dared not ask about, ones we did not know.

Every year after that, when we drove through that town, I was awake. Wide awake. I would peer out the window and look at every single woman on the street thinking, "That could be my mother, that could be my mother, that could be my mother." I wondered and wondered, "What does she look like? Does she have dark hair like me? Does she have skinny legs? Does she like sports? How old is she?" In fact, after that I started wondering these things no matter where I went. Every woman I passed in the street with dark hair became a face I projected my questions onto. I felt like the bird character in the book *Are You My Mother?*

There were so many women with dark hair, she could have been anyone. The idea of who she was and where she was haunted me and was in my mind constantly everywhere I went. It felt overwhelming to think that I may never find her. It instilled a deep determination in me from a very young age to search for her and to find the answers to these questions.

I remember thinking very early on, "I wonder if she is overweight and wears thongs," with a deep dread in my stomach. Already the conditioning of a lesser woman was installed in me. The father I was given was a misogynist. All women were referred to by the way their body looked and the way they dressed, not by who they were as people. The message that the worthiness of other women and my own worthiness is based on how my body looks, my weight and how I dress was deeply embedded in my psyche and is one I'm still learning to unhook from.

My strongest memory growing up was crying myself to sleep night after night wondering where my mother was, who she was and if she longed for me the way that I longed for her. In fact, I pretty much convinced myself that she was young, very young, and therefore she could not keep me. It never occurred to me that she did not want me. I vowed to myself that I would find her as soon as I could. As soon as I turned 18, I would search for her and we would be reunited and it would be sunshine and lollipops and we could be back together again, just the way we were meant to. I used to imagine that she would tell me with tears in her eyes just how much she was sorry and that she missed me and thought about me every day the way that I did about her. I was so ready to forgive her, in my eyes she was the victim of a terrible circumstance that kept us apart.

When I finally did turn 18, I was already a mother myself. My son was exactly one month old and the greatest love of my life. There was no way in the world that anyone would take my baby from me or that I would give my baby to a stranger. He was mine, and mine forever. This only reinforced my fantasy that my mother had her baby forcibly taken from her.

The questioning about who she was and therefore who I was grew stronger and I wanted answers. At 21, I finally told a close friend of the never-ending thoughts in my head that I had never spoken out loud before in my life ... that I wanted to find my birth mother. She encouraged me and I made some phone calls and ended up with my Original Birth Certificate. It had my mother's name on it. I finally got to see and say her name. It felt like magic in my mouth. Like a sweet butterscotch I could keep on my tongue and savour for a long time.

I didn't know where to start my search. My friend suggested I try the phone books in the library. I had thought of this already but felt the chances of finding her seemed impossible. I was sure she'd be married by now and had changed her name. I tried some birth, death and marriage searches first but came up with nothing, so I took myself off to the local library one day and searched through every single phone book until finally I found some folk with the same surname. I made some phone calls and finally got her phone number.

Meeting my mother was like putting the final jigsaw piece in a puzzle in some ways and like opening the door of an airplane when it was in full flight in others. She was beautiful. She had dark hair like me. She was intelligent. We could talk for hours. We looked alike. We ordered the same food off the menu. We drove the same make and colour of car. We wore the same glasses frames. We were interested in the same things.

Eventually, after all of the falling in love had subsided and settled, knowing she could do no wrong in my eyes, I was ready to receive some answers to the myriad of questions I had. And this is where the fantasy eroded. This is where my innocence was taken advantage of. This is where the lies started. This was the beginning of having my heart shattered.

I have no doubt that my birth mother did love me as the baby she relinquished, but she did not like me much as an adult. She was jealous of me being a mother. She did not like the way I was raised and the values of those who raised me. She was 18 when she fell pregnant and did not want to keep me. She never apologised. She could not see my pain. She lied to herself and to me numerous times about who my father was. She hid the truth and the story of what had happened and who she'd been intimate with. As a result, I missed out on a decade of vital time in relationship with my paternal family. Again, she never apologised. I spent two whole decades receiving random middle-of-the-night drunken texts from her. I had to block her numerous times.

Getting to know my birth mother was bittersweet. I feel sad that we didn't get the happy-ever-after fairytale ending. However, despite being in reunion for over two decades and now being estranged, I don't blame her. I see her pain and I forgive her, and I'm learning to forgive myself for all the ways I've self-abandoned. Adoption is not natural. How could any of us have the skills to navigate such complex loss and the consequences of such loss?

Contacting My Mother

My heart pounded like a drum beat in a heavy metal band. It beat so hard I could hear it from the outside in, as I stood in the corner of my kitchen. Sweat tingled through my hands and fingers like an electrical current. I was 21 years of age and had moved out of home with my three-year-old to live independently from my parents a year before.

I held the phone in my shaking hand, all noise around me now disappeared into the background. The dial tone, the only sound I could hear, getting louder and more insistent with each ring. Mouth dry, hands now dripping. Waiting, waiting. "C'mon. Pick up. Please?"

Several months earlier I had received my Original Birth Certificate in the mail. I remember seeing her name in print for the very first time: *Julie H.* So foreign to me, I had to repeat it over and over and over again until it was seared into my brain like a freshly branded calf. Branding is a technique for marking livestock so as to identify the owner. Surely if I repeat her name enough we will be bonded right?! She will be mine and I will be hers?

Once I had her name, I naively thought it would be easy from there. Now that I knew her name, now I could finally find her. I'd waited my whole life to find her. I waited like a child waiting to be picked up after school. I was ready, bag over my shoulder. Waiting at the gate eagerly, watching like a hawk as each child's parent came and went. She never came though, so I took on the job of finding her. At first, I set about doing a death search and a marriage search in the state I lived in. Both came back with nothing. So, I knew she hadn't died in Queensland, or been married there either. "This is going to be a bloody long and expensive search if I have to do two searches in every state" I thought. It felt impossible. She could have moved overseas.

Feeling stuck, I gave up for a while. Eventually, I dragged myself along to the local town library to search the endless shelves of phone books. I sat on the floor between the shelves of books by myself, like a child in the school halls at lunch time hoping not to get caught. One by one, state by state, pulling out phone book after phone book. A couple of hours went by, getting more and more disheartened as I opened and closed book after book. Finally, the last state, Western Australia. My finger slid tentatively down the page under the letter 'H'. There it was. There it was. Her name. She wasn't dead. She wasn't married. My hands shook as I wrote down the number on an old piece of scrap paper I found in my bag. I scrambled to my feet like a newly birthed foal, legs wobbling trying to find ground.

That was a week ago. Finally, with as much courage as I could muster, I was ready to make the call.

"Hello, Julie speaking" her voice softly sang down the line.

"Hello, we have not met, my name is Monique, I was born at the Nambour Hospital in Queensland. The name given to me was Norel Veronica." Pause. Heart pounding.

I had rehearsed that line over and over and over again like the rotations on a record player. I don't remember what came next. It's all a blur now, but I do know that we talked for over an hour. We talked like parrots at sunset, and by the end we had decided that she was coming to visit. She was going to fly from Perth all the way to my hometown in Central Queensland to meet me, for the first time in 21 years. I was elated.

I could breathe again. Whilst my mind raced, my body softened for the first time in two decades. I was finally going to meet her. My mother. I was going to see what she looked like, hear her voice again, watch her move, read her face, find out 'why.' The burning unanswered question inside ... why?

My Brother Tony

My brother Tony died 18 months ago. He was 49 years of age. My age now.

My brother Tony was my older brother. He was my adopted brother.

My brother Tony was a sensitive child. He was in love with animals and the natural world.

My brother Tony was kind and loving. He loved me so much throughout my whole life.

My brother Tony was teased and bullied throughout his childhood.

My brother Tony came out when he was 18. He endured the painful rejection and taunting of our misogynist and homophobic adoptive father. He endured the continual deaths of so many friends during the AIDS epidemic in the 80's. He endured the loss of his one and only partner by suicide. He endured the pain of never knowing his biological family.

My brother Tony was sexually abused by the same family member who abused me. In my early 20's I told my family I had been sexually abused by my older cousin throughout my whole childhood. When my brother Tony spoke about having the same experience, he was not believed, he was gaslit. I was sent to question him, to see if he was telling the truth. After all, he was the 'dramatic' attention-seeking one. It didn't matter that everything we talked about corroborated our stories. It didn't matter that I told them he was telling the truth.

It never mattered to my adoptive parents. We were always at fault. It was in our genes apparently.

My brother Tony was addicted to hard drugs in his 20's. He spent a decade selling his body for love and money.

My brother Tony was addicted to alcohol and weed in his 30's and 40's. He told me that he intended to live hard and die young. He said he wanted to die by the age of 40.

My brother Tony accessed his Original Birth Certificate when he was in his early 30's. He wanted to find his birth mother. He had all sorts of fantasies about her. He looked up her name and found an address near where we lived and he drove by the house over and over again, but never daring to go in, or to make contact to see if in fact this was indeed his mother's house.

My brother Tony was tortured by the fantasy of her and longed for the reality of her.

My brother Tony was told by my adoptive father that she would never want to meet him. That his life was a mess, that he would disrupt her life, that he wasn't enough and that he needed to pay off his debts and clean himself up.

My brother Tony died that day. On the inside. I watched him plunge deeper into the pain and abyss of addiction. He kept trying so hard, to be better, to do better, to be what Dad wanted him to be. It was an impossible task.

I found it hard to watch. I didn't know what to do. I started to distance myself. His trauma was deep. His addiction was deeper. I was busy raising my children, building my career. All the while I was building, he was crumbling. Alone with no understanding of what was happening. He was loyal to my adoptive parents. He kept going back no matter how many times they fought with and gaslit him. They always looked like the heroes and he always looked like the failure.

Until one day at 49 years of age, my brother Tony left. He bought an SUV, packed up his beloved pets and ventured off around the country with a terminal illness.

My brother Tony was diagnosed with an illness that was related to his biological heritage. There was a slim chance that it would lead to death, but in his eyes, he was terminal and dying. In my eyes, he was drinking himself to death and would do anything to be connected to his biological heritage, even it meant his own demise.

The last few years were difficult to watch. Phone calls were long and meandering complaints and accusations. They were full of stories of relationships gone wrong. He would shift from joy to anger to deep grief and anguish all in one phone call or visit. His Facebook feed was full of endless posts every day, varying from saving pets from cruelty to racist right-wing slander.

He reached out to me over and over again. I ignored his reaching over and over again. I told myself I was too busy. I didn't have time. The truth was I didn't know what to do. It was so hard to see him in so much pain and knowing his death was imminent I did not know what to do. I didn't have an understanding of the toxicity of my adoptive family and their narrative about us. I did not yet have an understanding of adoption trauma.

My brother Tony died in March 2020 of a heart attack, alone in his small flat halfway across the country where he hoarded and drank himself to death. He died of a broken heart. I wasn't there, by his side, like he had always been by mine.

Dear Adoption

Dear Adoption,

You are heartbreaking. You broke my heart. Taking me from one mother and giving me to another woman and calling her my mother was just plain wrong. I did not know what had happened. I did not know what to do with the sadness, the grief, the anger. I was not allowed to cry, to rage, to question. You were supposed to do what was best for me and you didn't. What was best for me was staying with my family, not being given to some random family and being told to forget where I came from. As if I would forget. I am not without instinct, without heart.

Even an animal that has been separated from its earliest imprints remembers. Whilst I am not a fan of reunion stories designed to hit at the heart but that subtly favour saviourism, I once saw a short documentary that became popular on Facebook about a lion cub that was raised outside its natural habitat by its human owners in London and then was freed into the wild as it reached full maturity. Years later, those human carers returned to greet the lion and even though it was now wild and it had been for many years, the lion ran toward them both nearly knocking them over with affection and joy. Whilst humans don't appear to imprint the way that animals do, we do attach similarly. I watched this reunion over and over and over again, crying, almost sobbing. It touched something deep inside me. At the time, I couldn't put words to why I was feeling so much emotion.

I guess I know now. A longing to be reunited. A longing to remember and to be remembered. A longing to be held without fear and caution. A longing to know that I mattered. A longing to show love with exuberance. The overwhelming emotion was an implicit awareness that our bodies remember those we fall in love with. And I did fall in love. I fell in love with my mother's heartbeat, her voice, her movement, her rhythms. She was my world and I was connected to her in every intimate way possible and you took that away. You broke a natural biological bond. You erased her from me and then pretended she didn't exist. As if that connection meant nothing, when it was everything. Everything I was uniquely supposed to have to help me thrive in this world.

My ability to reach for love was suspended. My ability to receive love was put on hold. The patterns we need to sustain love in later life were interrupted. A baby is meant to feel satiation; to take in nutrition, touch, sustenance, eye gazing, and smell until it permeates every cell and sends the message, "you are welcome, you are wanted, you are adored, you are loved." This receiving is paramount to later being able to be seen, to feel enough in the eyes of others and to then being able to reciprocate and give love, care, and help from a place of worthiness. Not from a place of need, or emptiness. This is the patterning I didn't get. This led to a life of ongoing heartache, misattunements, being lied to, being cheated on, staying when I should have left, leaving when I should have stayed. Endless searching for love. Endless beginnings and endings. Never feeling satiated. Never feeling safe enough to really be myself.

The blatant disregard for this human right, to stay with my mother; to be held, touched, seen, nursed, rocked, soothed, loved by my mother, has impacted my whole entire life. I was unable to bond with my carers. They fed me, clothed me, housed me, made personal sacrifices and paid for my initial education. These are no small thing, and I appreciate I was given a sense of family. However, they never once told me they loved me. They did not touch me with any kind of affection. They did not look at me with adoration in their eyes. They did not protect me from family predators. They did not guide me nor inspire me to be the best person I could be. They did not securely attach to me or me to them. Yet they expected loyalty, respect and trust from me as their daughter. They expected me to play their game of gratitude and lies, to pretend I was someone I was not, to stay with them and be grateful to them forever, to be like them no matter what, to have the same values and opinions, and to never become different from them. In other words, they did not want me to be my inherent, authentic self. To have interests and values that differed from them that were valued and valuable. They cared for me, but they neither liked me nor loved me sufficiently.

Although I played your game for four and a half decades, deep down I knew things were wrong. I never forgot. I felt displaced, like a square peg in a round hole my whole life. Throughout my childhood, other adults would often comment on my sad face, and ask what was wrong. The truth is that I tried to love them, but I just didn't even like the people that I was supposed to be learning the most fundamental lesson in life from: how to love and how to be loved. How can you learn this deeply wired-in biological need for love, from people you don't feel a connection with? From people who don't even see your broken heart, let alone acknowledge it? Who doesn't see or value your unique differences? Who, in fact, feels threatened by who you are, where you've come from and who you may become?

Adoption, you broke my heart, but you did not break my spirit. You were a practice that did a great deal of harm. Whilst you happened to me and are a part of my story, you are not who I am. I do not take you on as my identity. Through my own seeking, my own strength and integrity, I have found that I am a strong biracial Australian indigenous woman. I now know my ancestors and feel how they guide me and give me strength. I am a woman with wisdom, fire, passion and warmth. I seek justice and fairness. My courage to face challenges with grace and dignity has evolved and I now see that I am loving and worthy of great love in my life. I am who I am despite you, not because of you.

My Flourish Experience

As both a professional psychotherapist and an adoptee, I had found a way to completely compartmentalize and keep separate my painful experience and voice as an adoptee from my professional persona and the way I presented myself to the world. This was kept neatly separated by the unspoken understanding that I was never to talk about Adoption in my family, mention it to anyone, or even think about it. I had read a lot of literature on the topic, having been through my first search and reunion as a young adult. I even worked in the field of Post Adoption as a counsellor and mediator. As a result, I was well versed on the issues of adoption. Yet at 49 years of age, I had never even spoken about my lived experience of my adoption in any kind of substantial way to anyone. It was killing me.

Making a commitment to attend a weekly writing group with other adoptees was ignited by the thought that I may like to write a book about my experience of adoption, something my adult sons could read one day to understand me better. I was articulate, I liked to write, I had two Masters degrees; it was something I thought if I just made the time, I could do. I soon learned week after week, that I had no words. That I had no language to speak about MY experience. I knew I had a lot to say, but each time I reached for the words to write I came up blank. For the first time in a long time, I felt inarticulate, rambling and as though I was just sitting on the surface, unable to touch the deeper well inside. I spent a lot of each session 'zoned out' and dissociated, missing a lot of what was being said in the group. I was way out of my comfort zone. I thought about quitting often.

As the weeks went on and I started to really listen to the voices of the other adoptees in the group, my heart was blown wide open. They were saying things that were heartbreaking, powerful, moving, shocking, angering, deeply unsettling, funny and at times strangely settling. They were saying things I'd never dared to tell anyone before. They were saying things I'd felt, but that I didn't yet have words for. I felt so inadequate that I couldn't describe my experience. I now know that the trauma of adoption is a complex one and starts with our relinquishment, a time when we have no language, and continues throughout childhood, when developmentally we have little understanding about what is happening to us. Of course I had no words, I had no way of making sense of what was happening inside me as a result of what had happened to me.

Over the year, beyond listening to one another read our writing, we began to reach out to one another outside of the group. We began to truly bond, with one another individually as we heard about what was happening in one another's lives, and as a group through social media and group chats. This sense of community and connection to other women who have experienced something as debilitating and life-long as adoption changed my life. I found a sense of family, a place of belonging. Women who would have my back no matter what. And I felt the same about them. I also started to find my voice. I started to speak up about adoption in public spaces. I had long and substantial conversations about my life and the impact of adoption with another member of the group who listened deeply and validated my experience with fervent understanding and attunement. My life started to make sense. These understandings were difficult to realise and painful to feel, however with the support and connection I felt from my community, I was able to grow through the unbearable realisations and truths that were coming to light.

It is my belief that we can't truly heal until we have told our story, in its entirety, and until we have been heard by someone who matters to us. I am deeply grateful for the experience of Flourish and the opportunity to find my voice and a shared sense of belonging.

Monique's Story:

I have known that I was adopted since I was about five years old. I was the youngest daughter and child in my adoptive family. I grew up with two older adopted brothers. I am the only child of my biological mother and the eldest daughter of three to my biological father. I have two biological half-sisters. I searched and reunited with my birth mother at the age of 21 and through DNA evidence found my birth father at the age of 30. I was relinquished at birth and adopted at six weeks of age through the Queensland Government in 1972, which was the height of the 'Forced Adoption Era' in Australia. Around 10,000 babies were adopted that year alone. My name on my Original Birth Certificate was a name my biological mother did not recognise. She wanted to call me Sarah after her Grandmother. I have kept the first name given to me by my adoptive parents which means 'advisor,' added the name of my paternal Aboriginal grandmother and my maternal great grandmother, and changed my surname to Pangari, which is an Aboriginal word that means 'of the soul.' I am no longer in contact with my adoptive family and have friendly but limited contact with members of my biological family.

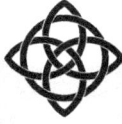

ROWAN DYER

CALIFORNIA

THE YEAR I SPENT IN FLOURISH was one of the hardest and best years of my life. In this group of adopted adults, I finally felt like I belonged, at age 59! I am filled with gratitude for the gifts I received from this group of amazing human beings. One of the best gifts was the gift of being seen and mirrored by the only people capable of seeing me for who I am – a woman who was given away at birth by her mother, and given to strangers. I am a singer, and in Flourish I experienced a new kind of singing that was deeply healing.

I told the group a story about my time with a young adoptee friend that I spent time with every week, so that she could know what it was like to be with another adoptee. When she was only five years old, there was a day when she was sad and agitated and unable to be calm. I asked her if she would like me to sing her a song and she said yes. I sang, "It's You I like" by Fred Rogers. I knew all the words which was something of a miracle! My young friend came over and put her head in my lap and listened quietly for the entire song. It was a time of connection and peace for both of us. After I told my Flourish friends this story, our leaders asked me to sing it right then. I did, even though I was very nervous and didn't think I would remember the words. I remembered the words, and the experience of singing to other adoptees, a song that says, "I see you, and I like you, all of you, right now," was something that helped heal my broken heart.

It became our tradition that I would sing it to each member on their birthday, or the day nearest it. Everytime, a stillness would come over our group and tears would flow freely. I am thankful for being able to experience seeing and being seen for the first time in my life.

I began having dreams of changing my name and my new name, Rowan, came to me in my dreams. I did not have anything against the name I grew up with, in fact, my previous name means "song"! But I didn't feel attached to my name in any way. I felt entirely neutral. But when I thought about the name

Rowan, I felt strong and connected and free. So in March, I created and led a ritual with my husband and son and some close (non-adopted) friends. We met outside under a tree at night on the Spring Solstice which would have been the time that I was conceived. It was a time of claiming myself and loving myself. I have decided to use my given name in my work and family world until my adoptive mother dies and then I will change my name legally to Rowan. When I am with my Flourish friends, who are my chosen family, I am Rowan. I am seen and loved and known. It feels good.

❖

Claiming Myself

Rowan's Name-change Ritual

20 March 2021

I was relinquished at birth in December of 1961.

I was given no name.

I was listed only as baby girl Wadsworth on a birth certificate that is legally hidden from me by the state of California.

I was adopted and named Carole Jeanne by the couple who adopted me.

My birth certificate was changed to say I was born to them.

I was loved by my adoptive family, but I never fit.

We did not vibrate at the same frequency. I never belonged.

I was not seen for who I was, a human being, born out of and into trauma.

Severed from my roots, disguised as another's child, never to know my origins, my people, my true identity.

Now, I claim myself.

I claim the power in naming myself, and the name I have chosen is Rowan.

I am in the process of finding my true nature in the shards and rubble of my past, of seeing where Rowan was throughout my life: hidden, but present and witness to my pain, my grief, my despair.

Rowan was and is my essence:

my love of connection,

my yearning to belong and to see myself mirrored in another,

my love for my family, given and chosen, especially Aidan and Thomas,

my love of community and music, and beauty,

my joy in singing, alone, and with others,

my desire to dance and be with the trees,

my prophetic voice demanding justice and healing

for all who are oppressed and exploited,

my love of water, of being in it, or in a boat, or just sitting near it,

my heart connection with animals, especially dogs,

my dogs Colette, Elke, Cecelia and of course, Mr. Bojangles,

my love of poetry and story and solitude.

There is great power in a name.

A name reveals one's essential nature,

so for me, this is a time of transition and a rite of passage,

a step toward claiming myself as no mother or family did.

I will mother myself and claim my authenticity and power.

This Is To Mother You by Sinead O'Connor (sung by Rowan, Aidan on guitar)

The Rowan tree has a long, sacred history.

In Celtic mythology it's known as the Tree of Life.

Since ancient times people have been planting a Rowan tree beside their home

for courage, wisdom and protection.

The Rowan tree embodies life, beauty, creativity and strength.

Aidan sings and plays *Riverman* by Nick Drake

As I take this name, may I grow deep roots that will nourish me, and may I let my branches be full and free and alive with the wind and birds and beautiful fruit. (Tom and Aidan place a stole around my shoulders).

As I continue to live and breathe and move and grow, may my branches be shade for my beloved family and friends. May I have strength to always work for justice for women and all oppressed people, and for the healing of Earth, our true mother.

Gentle Arms of Eden by Dave Carter (sung by Tom, Aidan plays guitar)

I invite my friends to give me their blessings at this time. (I receive six blessings.)

I give thanks for everything that brought me to this time of claiming myself and my name. I yearn for connection, for belonging and for mutuality. I dream of dancing under the stars with my people, and singing, and laughing, and sharing wonderful meals. Thank you for sharing this time and for holding space with me.

I love you,

Rowan

Rowan's Story:

I was relinquished in Santa Ana, California on December 20. Four days later, on Christmas Eve, I was brought home by my adoptive family. My four-year-old brother, Andrew, held me in the car on the way home. My mother said that the hospital wouldn't let her hold me until she was legally allowed to take me home, so the only touch I received for the first three days of my life was when the nurse would feed me from a bottle or change my diaper. I experienced the trauma of being separated from my mother, the only world I had ever known, and then left alone in a plastic box in the hospital nursery with no loving gaze, with no mother's milk, no arms to hold and protect me. This is a trauma that should never be inflicted on any human or animal. My mother made it clear that my adopted brother and I were not allowed to tell people that we were adopted. And when I did tell my childhood friends, my mother was furious and didn't speak with me for days, as she often did when she was angry at me. I developed an ulcer on my vocal folds in my twenties and realized this was a direct result of being silenced and not being allowed to tell my story, and not being seen. I spent my life feeling invisible, even as I had many wonderful friends and a successful career as a choir director and singer.

I did DNA testing five years ago and found the name of my birth mother who was already deceased. My birth father is one of three brothers but so far I don't know which one. I have no information about my ancestors or family history. I have never known the feeling of being mirrored by a parent, sibling, aunt, uncle or cousin. My son is my only biological connection to this earth and that connection has saved my life on many occasions when I felt so much pain that I wanted to cease to exist. I dream about finding relatives who knew my mother and father, learning stories about my people, and seeing myself in other humans. My work now is to love myself, to mother myself, to choose myself. I am the only one who can.

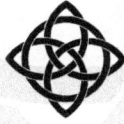

RUTH MONNIG

Flourish, For Me

WHEN I JOINED, what I really wanted was a group of people, or a "someone," to tell me how I was supposed to cope with the fact that my birth mother lives less than a mile from me and wants nothing to do with me. That didn't happen. My mother still lives down the street, still thinks I am the ruin of her life, and we have still never met, nor have I ever consciously seen her. All of those feelings of horror I had when I joined, are still, for the most part, there.

In the world of my own discomfort, I got something I didn't expect. Something that is infinitely better. A group of someones who understand my dilemma. A group of soulmates who don't need any explanations and who won't look at me, glaze over, and say, "Will you ever just get over this?" They know I won't, and they are simply there to hold my hand while I feel. They expect nothing from me but presence. In a world in which I sometimes can't function, for them, I show up. And they show up, too.

I know everyone's first name. Some of us have changed names over the year. I can't say I know everyone's last name, or everyone's profession or relationship status I have only met three of them in person. The last two I met both told me I was taller than I appeared on calls. I don't know eye color, or favorite color, or anything else surface purposeful, but I know them more intimately than most people I have ever known. We could have a totally silent Zoom call and every single one of us would likely have a pulse on how each feels just by reading a face or a glance. A silent meeting, in this group, might have a few tears, but more likely, it would devolve into gales of laughter. We all just get it, and each other.

You know that feeling, when you go to a party that you don't really want to go to and you search the room for someone safe? You know how relieved you feel when you see that person whose presence will make the whole experience tolerable? I look at each of these people, and can imagine seeing each one and saying, to each, "Thank God you are here." Being in a room with any of them would make me feel peace.

How often do you have a group of twenty-five people in your life you would take a bullet for? Remember, we have never met in person. We live everywhere. Two live in Australia. We have folks from sea to shining sea. California has a handful up and down the coast. Hawaii. Washington State. Montana. South Dakota. Colorado. Arizona. Oklahoma. DC. Florida. North Carolina. New York. Massachusetts. I am probably forgetting a few but it doesn't really matter. Where they are is irrelevant. I know they are there for me, wherever "there" is.

This is a group of people with whom I can say, on any given day, "My sense of despair is so great, I don't think I can live." I can also say things like, "It would be OK if my mother had chosen to abort me." They will be the ones who understand, who know there is no need to call 911, and know that I am speaking the truth without drama. I don't have to explain anything.

When someone is down, or has a story to tell, we are there, via the magic of Facebook, with basically real time support. It is rather astonishing. We are there because they are there and we all can relate to the feelings we can't describe to others.

We are quirky, creative, honest and loving. Some people are teary ... for every reason. Others are strong and stoic. The whole group has a certain sense of humor that should be bottled for PLU (People Like US). People are at different stages. Some are in reunion, some are doing DNA testing, some have had secondary rejection, some, well, all, are living while adopted.

We have seen people transform. They even look different. One of them was seriously shy and suffering. She is an artist with a complicated family and complicated emotions. Over the weeks her face changed. Her voice changed. She went from sad girl to strong, strong, STRONG woman. Another went through DNA testing, search angel assistance and ultimately a very positive reunion with both parents. Her posture is different. Her voice is stronger. Her face radiates. She is clear. It is astonishing.

Many of us write. Many of us are artists. Some of us have a knack for the one-line pun that would turn an interpretive dance into a tap dance. We are pet owners. Zoom frequently features a canine companion. Children, occasionally, too. Some are parents. Some are therapists and caregivers. Some are spouses. Some of us are runners. Others paddle and hike. We really are all over the place. It is hard to say if, in another setting, we would have gravitated toward each other.

I think the universe would have brought us together one way or another. We share an otherness not known to many. There is no other group I would rather, "other," with. Two of us fell in love with each other. I fell in love with a group. We have been seeing each other for a year. My mother, down the street, wouldn't approve. But this is my choice. She didn't give me one. We will always be going ...steady.

RUTH'S STORY:

I was raised with a brother. He was also adopted, no relation to me. He is three years older and we are estranged. I am in reunion with each of my birth families, but not with my mother. My birth father died in 1986 and my birth mother wants no contact. I have a lovely relationship with aunts, uncles and cousins on both sides. I was relinquished at birth. I was adopted at two months of age. I always knew I was adopted. Lutheran Family Services was the adoption agency. I was not named at birth My adopted name is Ruth Jaye Monnig I have a biological half sister on my paternal side. She is 11 months younger. I was 50 when I searched for and had reunion with my biological family members.

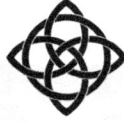

SHANNON

U.S.A.

Identity Revealed

I AM A LATE-DISCOVERY ADOPTEE, or LDA. I was a college student at home for the summer when I received a phone call from a woman who said she was my mother. I told her that she had the wrong number because I wasn't adopted. The woman proceeded to confirm details about my birth. She knew the hour and the hospital. The remaining details of the conversation were a blur; my head was spinning and I felt nauseous.

Shortly after, I heard my adopted mother and our house guest return home. I asked my mother to join me in my bedroom where I asked her about the phone call, expecting her to put my doubts aside so that I could start feeling the ground beneath my feet again. Instead, my mother raged, "You call that bitch back and tell her to go to hell and stay out of your life!"

Everything changed in that moment. I felt like I was floating and there was nothing to anchor me. In an instant, the key people in my life - my family - became strangers. There were no explanations, nor any concern about how this might affect me. My questions were met with more rage and demands that I keep quiet.

Suddenly, nothing in my bedroom belonged to me because I wasn't myself anymore. Everything belonged to another girl who had been worthy of being kept by her mother. Those new pink Polo tennis shoes that I was excited to wear were not mine. Nothing was. I was a throw-away, inferior to everyone around me. I haven't been the same since. The experience drained my energy and I've had to use every bit that is left to keep up and keep going.

Later that day, my mother told me that it was almost time to head to the restaurant for a family dinner with our guests, and that I needed to get dressed and freshen my face and to smile and to not dare speak a word to anyone of the revelation that had just shattered me. At the dinner table, my thoughts raced. I wondered who knew the truth. Our guests? My stepdad? My brother? Oh, and was my brother adopted? Were we related? We couldn't be because he looks like our parents.

The fact that he looked like my parents while I didn't and that he was favored over me so often suddenly made sense. I had always felt that for some reason I wasn't enough for my family. I'd spent my childhood and teen years wondering why I was so different and difficult and disappointing, and now I knew why. I was adopted when my mother thought she couldn't have a child of her own. Then she became pregnant almost immediately. I don't share any DNA with my adopted family. We have never had the chemistry and familiarity that I witnessed them enjoy with each other.

Thirty years later, things haven't changed much. My adoptive mother still wants full control over the narrative of who her daughter is. I'm shamed for not hiding the fact that I'm adopted, shamed for having questions and feelings about my story, shamed for wanting to have a relationship with my birth mother, shamed for buying books and connecting with others and learning all I can to try to heal myself. The few discussions we've had about adoption have focused on her feelings and how she was betrayed. It seemed suffocating. I couldn't help but to pull away from her for my self-preservation. I began to avoid her and call only when necessary. She was offended by my lack of attention and recently asked me with disgust, "Do you think you are a good daughter?"

I feared if people knew the true depth of my pain, it would scare them away, and so I learned not to show pain or ask for help. I wasn't my own person; I was my adopted mother's person. I was teased and scolded for the separation anxiety – a natural response to relinquishment – that I experienced when I was younger. I spent so many years behind a mask, trying to please and comfort others. It was exhausting. I felt like something was very wrong with me.

A memorable Flourish writing prompt was to pretend that we were using a magic typewriter, and that what we wrote would come to fruition. The sky was the limit. I wrote:

I will heal myself physically.

I will nourish my body.

I will love myself.

I will grow my capacity to love and forgive others.

I will speak my truth and tell my story.

I will not be fazed by those who are skeptical.

I will help my son and daughter understand generational trauma and overcome the past. I will see them whole, both physically and mentally.

I will advocate for adoptees.

I will manage my grief and trauma like a boss.

I will love with abandon and be loved.

While these statements may seem simple, I could not have confidently penned this a year ago. It would have felt selfish, but I am learning that it is self-love. The relationship with my adopted mother is just one issue that I have addressed. There are many trauma issues that I want to open myself to examining and healing. While I have a lifetime of work to do, thanks to the support of my adoptee friends, I'm closer to living a bigger life, on my terms. Learning to protect my comfort, say no, and set boundaries is so incredibly difficult for me yet also intoxicatingly liberating. I am taking up more space and I'm less apologetic. I have as much right to live as anyone. I deserve full ownership of the rest of my life and I must soak up the pleasures of what is left. I want to begin flourishing!

SHANNON'S STORY:

I was relinquished at birth; one week later I was taken home by my adoptive parents. I was not given a name at birth. I was later given the name Shannon in my adoption which was handled privately by an attorney. I was raised with a brother who is biological to my adoptive parents. I am a late discovery adoptee – I learned my true identity at age 20. I am currently estranged from my adoptive family. I am in reunion with my birth mother and her family. I have experienced secondary rejection from my biological father. Being adopted is the most challenging issue I have faced in my lifetime.

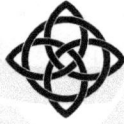

SUSIE STRICKER

MARYLAND

Community: A Place of Belonging

IT'S HARD TO CONNECT to the world when you never feel you are exactly where you are supposed to be. For so long, my home has been in the sadness of unbelonging. I was robbed of my autonomy when I was adopted. I live in a world where I am never seen nor fully embraced for who I am.

When I was adopted, I traded in honesty and wholeheartedness for safety. It's as if everything is temporary. My lack of trust has me living in constant discomfort from carrying all the heavy armor of the false self which exists to protect my true self from further harm. Protecting my true self from accessibility ultimately manifested in me as a constant state of hypervigilance. Living in constant hypervigilance is exhausting!

In 2014, after I laid the wooden box holding the ashes of my adopted mother next to where my adopted father was laid to rest in our church cemetery, I found myself feeling as if I was drifting out into open water. At the age of 50, I was so exhausted from years of being hypervigilant and I was tired of constantly swimming against the current. I had experienced grief and loss before. What I was experiencing and feeling was inexplicable and, in my mind, abominable. I had no words for it. I thought something was very wrong with me. I couldn't name what I was feeling. I was drifting into deep water where I could no longer see the shore and had no compass. My adopted parents' happiness was my North Star. They were my compass. They held the wheel while I rode shotgun. Now, no one was steering me in the direction they wanted me to take. Now what? I was lost and scared. What I was feeling almost felt ... familiar?

So, I did something I have never done before. I asked for help. It took me a few years to finally find the right therapist. However, I still didn't feel fully seen and understood. I still felt disconnected. Since my reunion with my biological family was not going as I had hoped and I experienced more rejection, I found myself searching for advice and support from other adopted people. That's how I found Flourish.

I don't know what I expected from Flourish. I guess I wanted someone to help me find out what is wrong with me. Who else would know better than a group of adoptees? I wanted to fix what was wrong with me and then be free from the pain, get over it and move on, just like everyone tells me to do.

I'm here to tell you that I did not get what I expected. I did not learn how to be free from the weight of pain forever. No one could promise me that I would no longer be afraid and everything was going to be easy from now on. What I got is something I never imagined.

What happened didn't happen overnight. It was a process. A journey filled with shared experiences of both struggles and victories. Over the course of the year, I struggled to connect. I held my cards close. I tried to impress and say and do the right thing. July rolled on by, the halfway point, and I found myself feeling disappointed. I couldn't give up now. I can't leave them, because that is exactly what I don't want to happen to me. I would be abandoning everyone. Besides, I can't go back to the way things were when I started. I had to keep going in order to Flourish.

The more I listened to other adoptee voices, the more I saw myself. Eventually it became clearer to me that, finally, this was a group of people who mirrored me. As an adoptee, I've never experienced being in the presence of a group of people who share many similarities. As our field of experience as a group expanded, I began to feel safe enough to allow myself to be vulnerable, because here was a group of people who showed me they had the capacity to hold space for me. Feeling encouraged to share and offering to provide the space to help me carry my pain, I found the courage to risk giving myself to the group. As I connected by reciprocating, the mirroring reflected back to the group. Furthermore, the accepting response to my contribution as a member of the group, left me feeling valued. I finally found a place where I belong.

I don't need fixing. What I need is a community. I need a space where the people are honest, patient, and continuously offer words of encouragement. I need a safe place where I can connect and experience the joy of friendship. By unlearning the unhealthy ways I respond to the world, the support of my Flourish community, a community of adoptees where I feel I belong, gives me courage to take ownership of my life. Every day I am encouraged to stop riding shotgun and to follow MY North Star by grabbing the wheel!

Letter to Humanity

Dear Humanity,

I need you to not mold me into something I am not. I need you to see me for who I truly am. I need the truth.

I need you to not blame my mother for the circumstances in which I was born into. Shaming is not the answer. I need you to have Compassion. Human beings should not be treated like transactions. I am not a clean slate that can be handed over as a band aid for an infertile couple. They are strangers. Adoption is not an event. It is my entire life.

My adopted family treat me as if I am their own, molding me so well that they say they forget I am adopted. I can never forget I am adopted. How can I forget that I am pretending that I am the child of two people with whom I share no DNA? Why must I pretend I am something I am not?

I beg you to let me live my truth. Let's all just agree that the social experiment failed. Let's just stop inflicting pain on innocent lives. Every child has the right to know their own identity and should never be denied the freedom to live their truth.

Sincerely,

Susie (originally known as Ellen)

Intro to a Book about Adoption and Play

This is a guide for all adoptees on how to act and speak unapologetically. Stop being in a constant state of hypervigilance. It's PLAY TIME! Time to get MESSY! Time to live YOUR life. Were you denied the privilege of self-love? Do you always feel you are never able to play your way? Do you ever feel that what makes you happy is not good enough for everyone else? Do you always act as a chameleon during play? Adoptees need to play in a way that is healthy for their true inner child. It's time to live a life of joy! It's time to KICK ASS! It's time to be free.

To soothe my inner child when my true self is struggling with the false self, I recall a fond memory of wearing my yellow slicker, with matching cap and galoshes, splashing through puddles (a favorite pastime) to the tune of "Raindrops Are Falling on My Head." I believe that memory remains so vivid because it was when I was feeling closest to my true self and I was free.

Dancing Toward True North

A popular analogy that is used to describe Life is by comparing it to a journey; The Journey of Life. I once came across a quote by Dr. Barbara De Angelis that describes the journey like it was a dance. "The journey between who you once were and who you are becoming is where the dance of life really takes place." Explorers often carry two tools while on a journey: a compass and a map. Every map includes a compass rose, highlighting North, giving the traveler the ability to read the map and a clearer understanding of which direction they need to go. The Celtic knot of journey forms into the shape of a compass rose depicting four points of direction, evoking the cycle of exploration and returning home.

After both my adopted parents passed, I experienced a grief so extreme I lost my sense of direction and purpose. I felt like I had just exited a wild amusement ride, totally discombobulated and disoriented. I no longer held the compass that pointed me in the direction of my adopted parents' happiness. They were now gone. I was engulfed in a fog of confusion. A voice was calling me, begging me to come out of the darkness. I realized it was the voice of my intuition, my original compass, pointing me in the direction of my true self.

As the deadline to submit my artwork quickly drew near, I pondered how to visually express my experience in Flourish. I love the image of self-discovery as a dance, giving the expression of being liberated. I envision our community dancing out of the fog as we speak and share our truth using our words and voices, guiding one another through the turmoil of loss toward our North Star, our true selves.

Susie's Story:

After I was relinquished at birth, I lived with a foster family until four months of age. At 11 months, my adoption, which was arranged through an agency connected to the Episcopal Diocese, was finalized and I was given the name Susan. Raised as an only child, I always knew I was adopted, but I didn't fully understand what it meant until I was around seven years old. At the age of 50, after both my adopted parents had passed, I contacted the state of Maryland's confidential intermediary services for assistance in my search for my biological family. I learned that I was the first-born child of both my unwed parents, who discontinued their relationship. I also learned that my mother had named me Ellen. By the time I met my mother, Alzheimer's had taken hold and she had lost every memory of me. Currently in my sixth year of reunion with my bio family, I have been through both positive experiences and quite a few disappointments as well. Due to the physical distance between us and life's daily challenges, my relationship with my father and my paternal siblings is progressing slowly. My first mother died a year ago and I currently have a good relationship with one of my three maternal siblings.

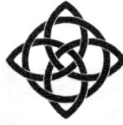

Flourish Monthly Themes

September 2020

October 2020

November 2020

December 2020

January: Belonging

February: Mutuality

March: Embodiment

April: Ownership

May: Health

June: Family

July: Truth

August: Dreams

September: Creativity

October: Play

November: Spirituality

December: Trust

September 2020

Trauma creates an attention vacuum greater than just an absence or longing for attention. We find a way to fill it to survive. What is your addiction? What happens to you in the liminal space as you reach for your addiction?

What do you do when there is too much of the right thing? How does that feel?

What happens when there is not enough of the right thing? How does that feel?

October 2020

What are three body sensations you have when you hear the words birth mother?

Write one sentence to your birth mother that is just right.

If you went into the heart place of you, what would it tell you to do tomorrow?

If your throat could talk, what would it say about when it feels open and when it feels closed?

What is the truest thing you could say to open your throat/voice?

What is the one thing you are terrified to say?

What was it like when you first fell in love? How did being adopted affect it?

Describe the romantic relationship between your adoptive parents.

What do you want from your future romantic life?

What small step could you take toward the future you desire?

November 2020

Describe your place at the holiday table when you were a child.

Describe your place at the table now.

Define what at the table means to you.

December 2020

List the traits of the person you want to become.

Describe a time when you were in your body and experienced hope.

Who does your body belong to?

Let your body write your story from birth to 6 years.

What is it like to look at your hand and realize it's been with you all along?

What graffiti would you write on the walls of your mother's womb?

What prayer words would you write on yourself, for yourself?

What touched you this year?

What things do you want for 2021 that feel challenging and are hard to see how you could achieve them?

What would you do with the extra energy that might come from removing all the energy-sapping entities from your life? What would you remove and what would you do with that energy?

January - Belonging

In a nutshell, who are you?

Why are you in this group?

Describe your first memory of feeling you didn't belong.

What was the fatal flaw that led to your relinquishment?

Where do you yearn to belong but don't know how?

Describe your experience of mutuality in your life.

Where and how do you find more opportunities for we in your life?

How can you belong when you don't know that you are real? What is real?

Describe your feeling of belonging in your family.

Respond to this quote from Brené Brown, *The Gifts of Imperfection*: "Because true belonging only happens when we present our authentic, imperfect selves to the world, our sense of belonging can never be greater than our level of self-acceptance."

Who am I? Who are we as contradictions? Who am I when I'm not adopting? What in me is not free?

February - Mutuality

Where are you hiding yourself in the group dynamic? What are you hiding and why?

What is important today in your life?

What comes up for you around mutuality? Where does it exist and where are you challenged with it in your life?

What risks are you not taking?

What risks are you going to start taking?

March - Embodiment

Draw your whole body. Indicate where you live in your body and the parts you are not even aware of.

What are a couple of pleasurable things you could allow yourself to do this week? What would it cost you?

Describe your experience of a recent event and how integrated (or not) your parts were (e.g., ecto, endo, meso).

Since the beginning of the year, is there something where you have been feeling more-ness?

What is something in your life where you might be encountering an upper-limit problem?

When you think about the erotic in your life, what comes to mind?

What is your experience of being an erotic person (e.g., emotion, devotion, or sexual) with other people?

How are you participating in the death of your juiciness?

When you reach for something from a state of longing, what do you reach for and what do you do with it?

April - Ownership

How are you not in 100% ownership in your life and how would you know if you were?

Where are you in ownership of your time, energy, and relationships and where are you not?

Tell the story of your North Star. What grand gesture could you/will you take to support it?

Are you living your dream? What is it? If you are not living it, what would it take?

Imagine yourself in the driver's seat of full ownership of your life. What kind of car is it? Who is in the car with you? What three things do you throw out the window? Where do you go first?

What song is playing?

How does your body feel if you give up fear, doubt, guilt and *shoulds*?

May - Health

In what ways are you taking care of your health to show up for Flourish?

What is important for you to share with the group today?

Write directions for the babysitter who is to care for you over the weekend as if you are the mother you needed.

Respond to the concept of the *nothing place* and the ways we adopt/adapt.

What are you participating in that is soul-sucking? If you became more grounded in the nothing place, what soul-sucking things could you release?

How would our lives change if we stopped bargaining with the *nothing place* and instead grounded into it? Does it change things if we find each other there?

Write about your experience with the *nothing place* this week.

How can being in the *nothing place* serve you? If it is a tool, what does it mean?

June - Family

Describe the experience of refusing false family versus opening to family that feels real. What risks are involved?

What would a *bright home* (David Whyte "House of Belonging") look like? Who is there?

What do you want to tell us about family right now?

How do we find empowerment for inner and outer concepts of family?

Write a *Dear Family* letter from before you were born. Tell your family what you will need to make your life go more smoothly.

Write a letter to adoption.

Assign a performance grade to family members.

What would it take to give yourself an *A* with your family? What would it take to earn an *A* from your family?

What would your life look like if you committed to only telling and living the truth for a year?

Pick one thing from the above and delve more deeply into it.

July - Truth

What has felt true to you? List things that have felt true in your life.

What is going okay in your life? What is not going okay?

What would you need/want in your day for it to feel, at the end of the day, like a satisfying, good day?

What would keep you from having those things in your day?

What is the truth of where you are in your life?

Describe the landscape there.

What is the truth of where you want to be and what does it look like there?

August - Dreams

Write a missing person's report about yourself using objective facts. Describe yourself.

Write *I Have a Dream* for the members of Flourish.

Draw our compass.

We lose our compass when we lose our mother.

How can I consciously create a compass in my body? Write about 3 of your dreams.

We were told our wanting was wrong, so it becomes heavy and a burden.

We have been cut off from our instincts (our mothers) so we don't trust our instincts.

What does dear sweet me want?

How do we stay soft and still investigate this very vulnerable and tender place while feeling alive, safe, and vital?

Walls and Dreams – we have dreams or wishes but then a wall comes up and keeps us from them.

The walls can come up and down.

September - Creativity

What is draining to us? What resources come naturally?

Return to wholeness – that's the healing.

We gave each other gifts.

We talked about SCOBY, necessary biproducts of each other. You need the mother but you don't want it in the final product.

Control is a substitute for trust – we gave each other more gifts.

October - Spirituality

Create and give a gift to your partner. Describe the gift.

What happens if you let in their gift for you?

What questions would you want to ask your birth mother?

Pick one question and describe what the answer would mean to you.

What do you do wholeheartedly? What things do you not go into wholeheartedly?

What were your adoptive/biological families' religious beliefs and how do you feel about them?

What gifts do you have to offer this community and what needs are satisfied by this community?

November - Spirituality

Write an introduction to the book entitled "Adoption and Play."

What are your needs from the group between now and the end of the year?

What is the most overused word related to your adoption story?

December - Trust

What is your relationship to trust in yourself?

Where are you starting to trust yourself in relation to others?

How has this year been a hero's journey for you? What have you let go of? What have you gained?

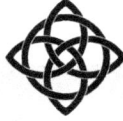

Other Resources for Adoptees

Inclusion does not imply affiliation to or endorsement of
The Flourish Experience

PODCASTS:
Browne, Louise and Reinhardt, Sarah (Hosts) *Adoption, The Making of Me* [Audio podcast].
https://adoptionthemakingofme.buzzsprout.com/

Davis, Damon L. (Host) *Who Am I Really* [Audio podcast].
https://www.whoamireallypodcast.com

Dinwoodie, April (Host). *Born in June Raised in April* [Audio podcast].
https://aprildinwoodie.com/the-podcast

Ghoston, Jennifer Dyan (Host) *Once Upon a Time in Adoption Land* [Audio podcast].
https://www.jenniferdyanghoston.com/once-upon-a-time-in-adopteeland-1

Holden, Lori (Host) *Adoption: The Long View* [Audio podcast]
https://www.adopting.com/adoption-podcasts/adoption-the-long-view

Marble, Heidi (Host) *Pulled by the Root* [Audio podcast].
https://www.pulledbytheroot.com/podcast

McDonald, Mike (Host) *The Rambler* [Audio podcast].
https://podcasts.apple.com/us/podcast/the-rambler/id1073467214

Radke, Haley (Host). *Adoptees On* [Audio podcast].

https://www.adopteeson.com

Shapiro, Dani (Host) *Family Secrets* [Audio podcast].
https://danishapiro.com/family-secrets/

Stanley, Ande (Host) *The Adoption Files* [Audio podcast].
https://theadoptionfilescom.wordpress.com

Online Groups and Websites

Adoptee Voices: Supporting Adoptee Storytelling. https://adoptee-voices.com

Adoptees and Addiction. https://www.adopteesandaddiction.com

Castro, A. *Adoption Mosaic.* https://adoptionmosaic.com (Resources for adoptees, birth parents, and adoptive parents).

McClintock, Reshma. *Dear Adoption: giving voice to those most affected by adoption: adoptees.* https://dearadoption.com

Grubb, Lynn. *Lynn Grubb: A blog about the adoption experience.*
https://noapologiesforbeingme.blogspot.com

howtobeadopted.com (Resources for adoptees, UK based).

Joy, Lora K. *My Adoptee Truth.* https://www.myadopteetruth.com (Adoptee blog).

National Association of Adoptees and Parents. https://naapunited.org.
(Conferences and resources).

Weatherford, Kirsten. *No More Misfit.* http://nomoremisfit.com
(Adult Adoptee Blog).

Nordine, Janet. MS, LMFT, RPT-S. *Experience Courage.*
https://www.experiencecourage.com (Therapist Adoptee Blog).

Pittman, L. *Adoption My Truth: A Fill-in-the-Blanks Life. 50 years in the making.*
https://adoptionmytruth.com (Adoptee Blog).

The Invisible Threads. https://theinvisiblethreads.com/ (LGBTQ Adoptee Blog).

Documentaries:

Hertzel, Michael and McClintock, Reshma. (Producers) & Alexander, Jeffrey and Vance, Sherie. (Directors). (2019). *Calcutta is My Mother* [Video file]. http://calcuttafilm.com

Sansom, Rebecca Autumn and Hawkins, Jill., PhD., (Producers) (2022) *Reckoning With The Primal Wound* [Video file]. https://reckoningwiththeprimalwound.com

Sunderland, Paul. (Lecturer) & LifeWorks: Dedicated to Recovery (Producer). (2011). *Adoption and Addiction: Remembered Not Recalled.* https://youtu.be/3e0-SsmOUJI.

Books:

No Author. (2021) *The Loving Parent Guidebook: The Solution is to Become Your Own Loving Parent. Adult Children of Alcoholics, Dysfunctional Families,* World Service Organization, Inc.

Barhydt, K.. (2020) *Dear Stephen Michaels's Mother: A Memoir.*

Breaux, V. and /Kilgore, S. (2020). *Rooted in Adoption: A Collection of Adoptee Reflections.* Book Baby.

Carroll, R. (2021) *Surviving the White Gaze: A Memoir.* Simon & Schuster.

Coles, G. (2006). *Ever After: Fathers and the Impact of Adoption.* Clova Publications.

Cordano, P. (2020) *10 Foundations For A Meaningful Life (No Matter What's Happened).* Balboa.Press.

Dana, D. (2021). *Anchored: How to Befriend Your Nervous System Using Polyvagal Theory.* Sounds True.

Easterly, S. (2019). *Searching for Mom: A Memoir.* Heart Voices.

Frankl, V. E. (2006). *Man's Search for Meaning.* Beacon Press.

Galbraith, M.C. (2021). *The Guild of the Infant Saviour: An Adopted Child's Memory Book.* Mad Creek Books.

Glaser, G. (2021). *American Baby: A Mother, a Child, and the Shadow History of Adoption.* Viking.

Grubb, L. (2015). *The Adoptee Survival Guide : Adoptees Share Their Wisdom and Tools.*

Hansen, R. (2013). *Hardwiring Happiness: The New Brain Science of Contentment, Calm, and Confidence.* Harmony.

Heffron, A. (2016). *You Don't Look Adopted.*

Heller, L. and LaPierre, A., (2021). *Healing Developmental Trauma: How Early Trauma Affects Self-Regulation, Self-Image, and the Capacity for Relationship.* North Atlantic Books.

Jakiela, L. (2015). *Belief Is Its Own Kind of Truth, Maybe.* Atticus Books.

Joy, L. K. (2021). *Goodbye Hypervigilance: Healing Adoptee Worry.* My Adoptee Truth.

Joy, L. K. and Foote, L. (2021). *NoBODY Looks Like Me: An Adoptee Experience.* My Adoptee Truth.

Joyce, K. (2013). *The Child Catchers: Rescue, Trafficking, and the New Gospel of Adoption.* PublicAffairs.

Levine, P.A. (1997). *Waking the Tiger: Healing Trauma.* North Atlantic Books.

Levine, P.A. (2015) *Trauma and Memory: Brain and Body in a Search for the Living Past: A Practical Guide for Understanding and Working with Traumatic Memory.* North Atlantic Books.

Lifton, B.J. (1995). *Journey of the Adopted Self: A Quest for Wholeness.* Basic Books.

Lockington, M. J. (2019). *For Black Girls Like Me.* Farrar, Straus and Giroux (BYR).

Lorde, A. (2000). *The Uses of the Erotic: The Erotic as Power.* Kore Press.

Mate, G. (2010). *In the Realm of Hungry Ghosts: Close Encounters with Addiction.* North Atlantic Books.

Mate, G. (2019). *Scattered Minds: The Origins and Healing of Attention Deficit Disorder.* Random House UK.

McDaniel, K. (2021). *Mother Hunger: How Adult Daughters Can Understand and Heal from Lost Nurturance, Protection, and Guidance.* Hay House Inc.

Monnig, R.. (2021). *The Keys Book: An Illustrated Story for the Adult Adoptee and the People who Need to Understand Them.* BookBaby.

Perry, B. and Winfrey, O. (2021). *What Happened to You : Conversations on Trauma, Resilience, and Healing.* Flatiron Books.

Poole Heller, D. (2019). *The Power of Attachment: How to Create Deep and Lasting Intimate Relationships.* Sounds True.

Richardson, J. (2022). *Dear Me .... Letters to Our Younger Adoptee Selves.*

Richardson, J. (2021). *Life In-Between: A Story of Adoption, Recovery and Connection.*

Rogers, F. and Flowers, L. (illustrator) (2020). I*t's You I Like: A Mr. Rogers Poetry Book.* Quirk Publishing.

Roszia, S.K. and Davis Maxon, A. (2019). *Seven Core Issues in Adoption and Permanency: A Comprehensive Guide to Promoting Understanding and Healing In Adoption, Foster Care, Kinship Families and Third Party Reproduction.* Jessica Kingsley Publishers.

Strauss, Jean A.S. (2001) *Beneath a Tall Tree.* Arete - USA Pub Co.

Trinder, E., Feast, J. and Howe, D. (2005). *The Adoption Reunion Handbook.* Wiley.

Turner, T. (2017). *Belonging: Remembering Ourselves Home.* Her Own Room Press.

Van Der Kolk, B. (2015). *The Body Keeps the Score: Brain, Mind, and Body in the Healing of Trauma.* Penguin Publishing Group.

Walker, P. (2013). *Complex PTSD: From Surviving to Thriving: A Guide and Map for Recovering from Childhood Trauma.* CreateSpace Independent Publishing Platform.

Webster, B. (2021). *Discovering the Inner Mother: A Guide to Healing the Mother Wound and Claiming Your Personal Power.* William Morrow.

Verrier, N. (2003). *Coming Home to Self: The Adopted Child Grows Up.* Verrier Publishing.

Verrier, N. (1993). *The Primal Wound: Understanding the Adopted Child.* Gateway Press.

Webb, J. and Musello, C. (2012). *Running on Empty: Overcome Your Childhood Emotional Neglect.* Morgan James Publishing.

Weatherford, K. (2021). *Finding My Way Home.*

Acknowledgements

Pam Cordano and Anne Heffron, for the idea of Flourish and their continuing effort in building connections with fellow adoptees.

Haley Radke, without *Adoptees On* none of us would have found each other, realized we were not alone and began creating new kinds of relationships.

The writers of this book that weekly entered Flourish to talk about the wounds of adoption and forge new friendships.

Diane Shifflett for the many hours she gave to editing and forming this book and who donated her time to the *Adoptees On* podcast.

The artists, Susie Stricker, Michelle Hinton, and Francine Bauer for the amazing artwork that is gracing the cover.

Vance at Crosscheck Design for the cover design and interior layout.

To the many adoptees we consulted on an array of topics to form this book, we could not have done it without your advice and guidance.

www.ingramcontent.com/pod-product-compliance
Lightning Source LLC
Chambersburg PA
CBHW022055020426
42335CB00012B/695